PUBLIC HEALTH IN THE 21ST CENTURY SERIES

FIREFIGHTER FITNESS: A HEALTH AND WELLNESS GUIDE

PUBLIC HEALTH IN THE 21ST CENTURY SERIES

Family History of Osteoporosis
Afrooz Afghani (Editor)
2010. ISBN: 978-1-60876-190-6

Cross Infections: Types, Causes and Prevention
Jin Dong and Xun Liang (Editors)
2009. ISBN: 978-1-60741-467-4

Health-Related Quality of Life
Erik C. Hoffmann (Editor)
2009. ISBN: 978-1-60741-723-1

Swine Flu and Pig Borne Diseases
Viroj Wiwanitkit
2009. ISBN: 978-1-60876-291-0

Biological Clocks: Effects on Behavior, Health and Outlook
Oktav Salvenmoser and Brigitta Meklau (Editors)
2010. ISBN: 978-1-60741-251-9

Infectious Disease Modelling Research Progress
Jean Michel Tchuenche and C. Chiyaka (Editors)
2010. ISBN: 978-1-60741-347-9

Firefighter Fitness: A Health and Wellness Guide
Ernest L. Schneider
2010. ISBN: 978-1-60741-650-0

PUBLIC HEALTH IN THE 21ST CENTURY SERIES

FIREFIGHTER FITNESS: A HEALTH AND WELLNESS GUIDE

ERNEST L. SCHNEIDER
EDITOR

Nova Science Publishers, Inc.
New York

NOTICE TO THE READER

LIBRARY OF CONGRESS CATALOGING-IN-PUBLICATION DATA

Schneider, Ernest L.
  Firefighter fitness : a health and wellness guide / Ernest L. Schneider.
      p. ; cm.
  Includes bibliographical references and index.
  ISBN 978-1-60741-650-0 (softcover : alk. paper)
  1. Fire fighters--Health and hygiene. 2. Volunteer fire fighters--Health and hygiene. 3. Health promotion.
4. Physical fitness. I. Title.
  [DNLM: 1. Health Promotion. 2. Occupational Health. 3. Fires--prevention & control. 4. Occupational
Groups. 5. Physical Fitness. WA 400 S358f 2009]

RC965.F48S36 2009
363.37092'2--dc22
                        2009031741

Published by Nova Science Publishers, Inc. ✚ New York

CONTENTS

PREFACE

This book highlights firefighting as one of the nation's most dangerous and hazardous jobs, with heart attacks, high physical stress levels, sprains, and strains all too common. Of all firefighters in the United States, 72 percent are volunteers. The leading cause of on-duty death among volunteers is heart attack. The leading cause of injuries for all firefighters is overexertion and strain. The prevalence of cardiovascular illness and deaths and work-inhibiting strains and sprains among firefighters illustrates the need for a comprehensive health and wellness program in every department. To address the issues specific to volunteers, the National Volunteer Fire Council (NVFC) developed this guide to health and wellness for volunteer departments and members. In 2003, the NVFC launched the ground breaking Heart-Healthy Firefighter Program specifically to address heart disease in the fire and emergency services. This awareness and prevention campaign targets all firefighters and emergency personnel—both volunteer and career. This is an edited, excerpted and augmented edition of a U.S. Fire Administration publication.

In: Firefighter Fitness: A Health and Wellness Guide   ISBN: 978-1-60741-650-0
Editor: Ernest L. Schneider   © 2010 Nova Science Publishers, Inc.

Chapter 1

INTRODUCTION

U.S. Fire Administration

EXECUTIVE SUMMARY

Firefighting is one of the Nation's most dangerous and hazardous jobs, with heart attacks, high physical stress levels, sprains, and strains all too common. Of all firefighters in the United States, 72 percent are volunteers.[1] The leading cause of onduty death among volunteers is heart attack. The leading cause of injuries for all firefighters is overexertion and strain.[2]

The prevalence of cardiovascular illness and deaths and work-inhibiting strains and sprains among firefighters illustrates the need for a comprehensive health and wellness program in every department. The fire service realizes that health and wellness programs benefit individual firefighters and the fire and emergency services as a whole; such programs can yield safer and more effective action by first responders to emergencies.

Many organizations have addressed the issue of health and wellness in the fire service. The National Fire Protection Association (NFPA) redeveloped its health and wellness standards in 2003. Since 1997, several career departments have worked with the International Association of Fire Fighters (IAFF) and the International Association of Fire Chiefs (IAFC) on a wellness initiative. To address the issues specific to volunteers, the National Volunteer Fire Council (NVFC) developed this guide to health and wellness for volunteer departments and members. In 2003, the NVFC launched the ground breaking Heart-Healthy

Firefighter Program specifically to address heart disease in the fire and emergency services. This awareness and prevention campaign targets all firefighters and emergency personnel—both volunteer and career.

Programs from across the Nation

In 2003, the NVFC State directors and alternates identified 16 volunteer departments with experience in health and wellness programs. The departments used many different approaches to health and wellness, including screenings, examinations, immunizations, education, behavioral modifications, and fitness programming. Fewer than half of the departments stated that their programs were well received, and 10 departments noted culture as an impediment to the program. The three greatest problem areas identified were lack of funding, lack of well-defined requirements, and the inability to keep members motivated.

As this Guide details, budget constraints should not be a major barrier to the implementation of a comprehensive program. Many opportunities exist to help reduce or eliminate costs, such as developing partnerships. The Federal Emergency Management Agency (FEMA) Assistance to Firefighters Grant program is especially effective; grants are available to establish or expand wellness and fitness initiatives for firefighting personnel.

Education is the best option to counter concern among members about increasing their time requirements. Understanding the risks and consequences of not participating in a health and wellness program is a critical step in creating and implementing a successful program. When presented with comprehensive reasons why they should participate, many individuals often do so.

In the 1992 version of this guide, nine programs were featured as case studies; in 2003, seven of these departments updated their program status, and three additional departments were studied. Six of the previously profiled departments are featured in the 2008 Guide. They served as models for other volunteer departments, and many of the programs featured continue to be viable today. Only one has been reduced substantially from its original scope. These case studies, as well as new ones, also look at how to implement different program components and address the concerns.

Developing and Implementing a Health and Wellness Program

Planning is the most important step in implementing a health and wellness program. A vision is needed to provide guidance on how to develop and implement an individualized departmental program. There is no model plan that will work for all departments in all places, but there are model elements and core components that should be implemented, including

- regular health and fitness screenings and medical evaluations;
- fitness program (cardiovascular, strength, and flexibility training);
- behavioral modification (smoking, hypertension, diet, cholesterol, diabetes);
- volunteer education; and
- screening volunteer applicants.

In a program where all of these components are combined, the volunteers pay more attention to their personal health and wellness, which will improve the department overall. If a department cannot implement the entire program at once, it is far better to initiate some of these components than to do nothing.

A priority to ensure the program is successful is to appoint peer coordinators. The coordinators should be the advocates and leaders for the health and wellness program within the department. The coordinators might come from a steering committee or be identified by the department leadership.

Once the components have been selected and the program implemented, health and wellness needs to be made a priority if it is to become a part of the volunteer fire and emergency services culture. When department leadership and health and wellness coordinators actively advocate participation (in both words and actions), volunteers will see that the department has identified health and wellness as a priority and will be more likely to participate.

INTRODUCTION

Firefighting continues to be one of the Nation's most dangerous and hazardous jobs, with heart attacks, high physical stress levels, and sprains and strains all too common. In the past 5 years, the fire and emergency services have focused their attention on overcoming these issues by working to change their culture. The NFPA has spent much time redeveloping and revamping its health and wellness standards, while career departments have been working with the IAFF and IAFC on a wellness initiative that began in 1997. In 2003, the NVFC launched the Heart-Healthy Firefighter Program, a heart attack awareness and prevention campaign that offers resources and support to fire and emergency services personnel.

Volunteer personnel face risks similar to career personnel when it comes to health and wellness. Yet the nature of member time constraints and tight departmental budgets in the volunteer service often inhibits the creation of comprehensive health and wellness programs.

Implementing a comprehensive health and wellness program could overwhelm the resources of many volunteer departments. Time, lack of program leadership, and insufficient funding pose serious challenges to most departments, which often struggle to deliver basic fire suppression capabilities.

This Guide provides the rationale and suggestions for implementing a health and wellness program successfully in the volunteer fire and emergency services. It also addresses many common roadblocks. The chapters are divided to help volunteer departments develop a program from the ground up:

- **Chapter II: State of Health and Wellness in the Volunteer Fire and Emergency Services** looks first at current causes for injuries and deaths among first responders. It then examines current health and wellness programs and initiatives, resources implementing and sustaining them, and why many programs have not been sustained.

- **Chapter III: Importance of Health and Wellness in the Volunteer Fire and Emergency Services** summarizes, in layperson's terms, the science behind major injuries and fatalities among first responders. This summary should provide motivation for firefighters and emergency personnel to engage in health and wellness programs.

- **Chapter IV: Volunteer Programs from Across the Nation** looks at actual health and wellness programs and trends in volunteer departments. It includes programs from the first and second editions of this Guide, as well as new programs that have been developed.
- **Chapter V: Development of a Health and Wellness Program for Volunteer Fire and Emergency Services Departments** gives a step-by-step guide to developing a health and wellness program in a volunteer fire or emergency medical services (EMS) department. The chapter discusses

common roadblocks faced by departments and other strategies to deliver a sustainable program.

- **Chapter VI: Implementing a Health and Wellness Program** brings together all of the recommendations presented throughout the Guide for developing a program.

This Guide ends with two appendices to offer more assistance with program development. Appendix A includes contact information for departments and resources, and additional references. Appendix B examines the relationship between cardiovascular risk factors and physical fitness.

End Notes

[1] Karter, Michael J., and Gary P. Stein. *U.S. Fire Department Profile Through 2006*. National Fire Protection Association, Nov. 2007.
[2] Karter, Michael, and Joseph Molis. "Firefighter Injuries for 2006". NFPA Journal, Nov./Dec. 2007.

In: Firefighter Fitness: A Health and Wellness Guide   ISBN: 978-1-60741-650-0
Editor: Ernest L. Schneider   © 2010 Nova Science Publishers, Inc.

Chapter 2

STATE OF HEALTH AND WELLNESS IN THE VOLUNTEER FIRE AND EMERGENCY SERVICES.

U.S. Fire Administration

Statistics show that firefighting is one of the most dangerous occupations in the world. Volunteer firefighter fatalities accounted for 73 percent of all firefighting-related deaths in 2006.[1] In that year, stress was the leading cause of onduty deaths among volunteer firefighters, leading to the death of 38 firefighters. Heart attacks were the direct cause of death in over 47 percent of onduty volunteer firefighter fatalities.[2] In both nature and cause, stress and heart attacks killed a higher percentage of onduty volunteer firefighters than career firefighters, making clear the need for increased emphasis on cardiovascular health, physical fitness, and overall wellness in the volunteer emergency services.

In 2007, the USFA reported 118 firefighter fatalities. About half of those deaths were volunteers. Almost 50 percent of these deaths were from heart attack.[3] These statistics underscore the health and wellness issues being addressed in this Guide, and show how current the problem is in today's volunteer fire and emergency services.

Many factors influence the occurrence of an injury, its severity, and its outcome. Without a doubt, the health of the individual sustaining the injury is one of the more important factors. Firefighting consists of periods of low activity punctuated by periods of intense, strenuous activity. Good physical condition is a critical component in the body's ability to transition successfully, without injury, between these two activity levels.

Undoubtedly, pre-existing medical conditions, including underlying medical conditions, as well as physical fitness, affect the health and safety of firefighters. The NFPA estimates that 83,400 firefighters were injured in the line of duty in 2006.[4] Many onduty deaths and injuries may have been avoided, or have been less severe, under the same conditions if there was no pre-existing condition.

Despite the known risks, thousands of volunteer firefighters and emergency medical personnel lack rudimentary medical evaluation and overall wellness that can ameliorate the physical stress of emergency response. According to the USFA publication, *Four Years Later-A Second Needs Assessment of the U.S. Fire Service*, only one quarter of the surveyed departments nationwide have a program to maintain basic first responder fitness and health, such as is encouraged by NFPA 1500, *Standard on Fire Department Occupational Safety and Health Program.*[5]

According to the study, a large number of firefighters serve as volunteers in smaller communities, where most fire departments do not have programs to maintain basic firefighter fitness and health. It is likely that implementing health and wellness programs in fire and emergency services departments could prevent or reduce volunteer injuries and deaths, since a body of evidence suggests that improved lifestyles reduce the risk of injury and death.

In 2008, the NVFC, in partnership with the USFA, completed a study entitled, "*Emerging Health and Safety Issues in the Volunteer Fire Services.*" This report provides information on initiatives, programs, and strategies for reducing fatalities among volunteer firefighters and emphasizes the importance of a structured personal health and fitness program.

OVERVIEW OF HEALTH CONCERNS OF VOLUNTEER FIREFIGHTERS

This section looks at the overall health concerns of volunteer firefighters and EMS personnel. A more detailed discussion of the benefits of a health and wellness program for firefighters and EMS personnel is provided in Chapter III. The discussion of health concerns is applicable to the fire and emergency services as a whole. The USFA death statistics are broken down by volunteer and career firefighters. Injury statistics encompass both collectively, and are not broken down by volunteer and career.

Cardiovascular Health

As shown in Figure 1, heart attacks are the leading cause of firefighter fatalities, accounting for 47 percent of firefighter line-of-duty deaths in 2006. The number of firefighters, both career and volunteer, who suffer heart attacks while off duty remains untallied. The physical demands placed on firefighters can be very high; they often must go from a state of deep sleep to extreme alertness and high physical exertion in a matter of minutes. Further, they must carry heavy equipment through intense heat while wearing heavy protective gear. While many Americans are at risk for heart disease, the nature of firefighting requires that firefighters be particularly careful in maintaining a high level of physical fitness to combat coronary problems.

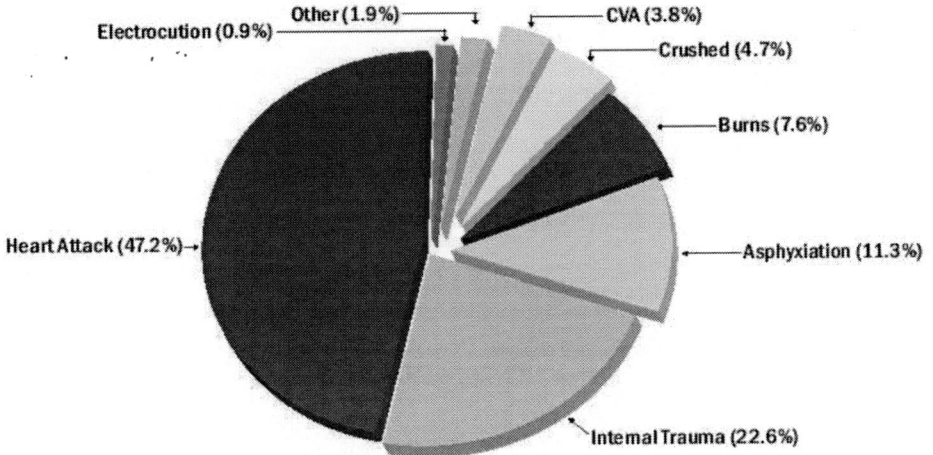

Source: United States Fire Administration. "Firefighter Fatalities in the United States in 2006," July 2007.

Figure 1. Fatalities by Cause of Fatal Injury (2006).[6]

The prevalence of heart attacks is a continuing problem. In 2006, "heart attacks were once again the number one cause of firefighter death."[7] *The USFA Firefighter Fatality Retrospective Study*: 1990-2000 analyzed the causes of more than 1,000 onduty firefighter deaths in the United States during the last decade of the 20th century and concluded that heart attack was the leading cause of death, accounting for 44 percent of firefighter line-of-duty deaths. Heart disease is also the leading cause of death in the United States, according to the American Heart Association.

The cardiovascular state of health and wellness in the fire service is of such concern that researchers identified a correlation to the public's safety. The high-risk profile for cardiovascular disease of firefighters should be a national concern.[8] Why firefighters should be concerned with cardiovascular disease and other risk factors is discussed in Chapter III.

Strains and Sprains

As shown in Table 1, in 2004, sprains, strains, and muscular pains accounted for 18.2 percent of overall firefighter injuries and was the leading cause of injury.[10]

Table 1. Firefighter Injuries by Nature of Injury.[9]

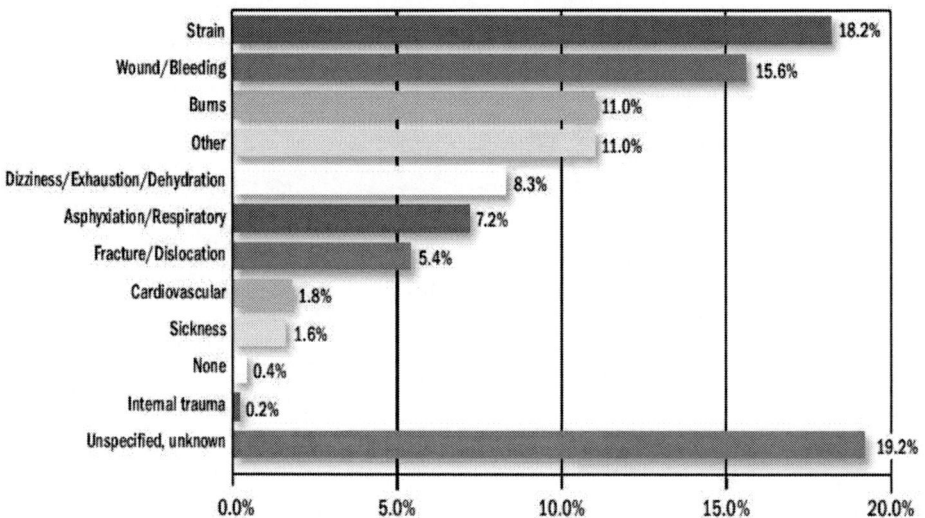

Source: United States Fire Administration. "Fire-Related Firefighter Injuries in 2004," February 2008.

In most injury cases, sprains and strains are caused by pulling, lifting, and carrying hoses; pulling or maneuvering hand tools and saws; pulling and lifting property or contents; lifting and moving ladders; and lifting other items. Very often, sprains and strains are exacerbated by preexisting conditions, called Cumulative Trauma Disorders (CTDs). CTDs, which fall under the umbrella term "ergonomic-related disorders," include tendonitis and nerve compression, conditions caused by continued, cumulative stress to certain joints, tendons, ligaments, and other body parts.[11]

Other sprains and strains can be worsened by back disorders, a frequent source of pain and complaint among firefighters, and another category of injury falling under "ergonomic-related disorders." Twisting, pushing and pulling, lifting, bending, and stretching can all cause such disorders, and even such a seemingly mundane action as continued sitting can be a problem. Regardless of the cause, pre-existing back disorders can result in more severe injuries among firefighters, especially in fireground situations.

Stress Levels

A majority of the job-related activities in the fire and emergency services can be characterized as sedentary, e.g., equipment maintenance, building inspections, or public education. Active firefighting, on the other hand, is a tremendously strenuous task. The firefighter can be taken from a complete resting state and within minutes be thrust into a dangerous, complicated environment where he or she is expected to perform at a demanding physical level.

Firefighters face a potentially deadly combination of stress, heat and high body temperature, and dehydration. Repeatedly placing such stresses upon an individual can take its toll. In stressful situations, such as a fire, researchers note that the body responds with a number of physiological changes. More adrenaline is released into the bloodstream, muscles tense, breathing quickens, and heart rate and blood pressure rise. Researchers also note, however, that fit individuals tend to take these physical responses in stride and with less wear and tear to the body.[12]

Weight Problems

In 2003, former Surgeon General Richard Carmona called obesity "the terror within, a threat that is every bit as real to America as the weapons of mass destruction."[13]

Dr. Stefanos Kales, MD, a Harvard researcher, led a study that analyzed data on all firefighter deaths between 1994 and 2004, except those linked to the 9/11 terrorist attacks. According to Dr. Kales, "We found that firefighters were generally very fit going into the service but over the course of a number of years—because of not exercising regularly, not eating right—many are becoming obese."[14]

An article in the *Journal of the American Dietetic Association* indicates that many overweight or obese firefighters may not even realize the potential problem.[15] Physical conditioning is crucial in public safety jobs because physical and emotional stress is unavoidable.

SUMMARY OF THE IMPORTANCE OF HEALTH AND WELLNESS

The importance of health and wellness and the need for developing and implementing health and wellness programs in departments can be summarized by the following 10 reasons:

Improves heart health. The importance of aerobic exercise cannot be overstated. Heart attacks cause the majority of deaths among onduty firefighters. Regular aerobic exercise helps prevent heart disease, strengthens the heart muscle, decreases clotting, and stabilizes the electrical activity of the heart. Aerobic exercise slows plaque buildup in the arteries and also helps to normalize blood pressure, especially in people whose blood pressure is somewhat elevated.

Improves heat tolerance. Exercise increases blood volume, which improves heat tolerance. Improved heat tolerance helps firefighters battle more intense fires.

Helps prevent Type II diabetes. Exercise improves the body's ability to regulate blood sugar, preventing Type II diabetes.

Reduces risk of strains and sprains. Physical activity strengthens the muscles and joints and other structures like tendons and ligaments that help hold the body together. This strengthening decreases the risk of strains and sprains—the leading cause of injury for firefighters.

May improve emotional state. Volunteer firefighters often deal with life-and-death situations when they respond to an emergency. Taking part in health and wellness programs improves their psychological and emotional states, which will improve emotional reactions during a life-and-death situation. An improved emotional state also improves self-esteem, self-efficacy, and sleep patterns, thereby reducing depression, anxiety, and stress.

Maintains weight loss. Exercise and proper nutrition help control body weight and are essential in any weight loss program. Weight loss is more likely to be maintained if a person continues to exercise. Weight loss increases stamina as well as aerobic abilities, both of which are needed for firefighting.

Maintains metabolic rate. By preventing the loss of metabolically active muscle tissue, exercise helps prevent the drop in metabolic rate that sometimes accompanies weight loss and the gradual decline in metabolic rate that occurs with aging.

Enhances ability to fight fires. Exercise can slow the loss of stamina, strength, flexibility, bone density, and metabolic rate, which all affect an individual's ability to fight a fire.

Prevents development of back problems. Maintaining flexibility in the muscles of the legs and lower back and increasing strength in the abdominal and back muscles can help prevent the development of back problems. Back problems among firefighters often develop from lifting hoses and equipment and moving apparatus.

Encourages overall healthy lifestyle. As fitness and nutrition improves, activity becomes easier. Exercise increases stress resistance and improves sleep. An active lifestyle also encourages other health-promoting habits, such as avoiding tobacco and alcohol and developing healthy eating habits. Besides feeling better, firefighters lower their risk for injury or even death with more and consistent exercise.

TOP REASONS WHY FITNESS PROGRAMS HAVE NOT WORKED

Despite the importance of health and wellness programs for the fire and emergency services, there are many obstacles to their inception and implementation. These obstacles must be addressed if first responder health is to be improved. Based on health advocate and former firefighter Michael Stefano's experience from administering a number of programs, the following are the five leading reasons for failure:[16]

Lack of information on risk to self. Many firefighters are not aware of the health risks of firefighting and, therefore are, uninterested in changing their condition. With many preventable injuries and deaths occurring annually, pertinent health information must be disseminated to motivate first responders to change their lifestyles.

Lack of individual goals. Programs that have failed to outline reasonable and specific individual goals are less likely to succeed. Program participants who feel they do not accomplish anything drop out. In developing any fitness program, the needs and wishes of the participants must be taken into account, and the participants must be able to see progress.

Lack of appropriate training. Fitness programs generally are not designed by professionals and thus lack the elements necessary for an effective program. While hiring a personal trainer may be too expensive for some volunteer departments, professional consultation should be sought to ensure the efficacy and safety of the program.

Lack of time to devote to the program. Volunteers already donate many hours to the fire and emergency services, and few feel they have excess time to devote to health and wellness. However, firefighter health is too important to ignore. Instead, fitness programs for volunteers should be designed around the members' personal and family time.

Lack of motivation. Even first responders aware of their elevated health risk choose not to participate in fitness programs. Lack of motivation is a serious challenge that must be addressed by each department. Chapter IV provides some suggestions.

OVERVIEW OF NATIONAL FIRE SERVICE WELLNESS INITIATIVES

The fire and emergency service's greatest asset is not equipment, apparatus, or stations, but rather its personnel. Through its personnel, departments serve the public, accomplish their missions, and are able to make a difference in the community. By committing to a wellness program, departments often increase their members' trust. This trust enhances every program and each call answered by the department. Placing a high priority on wellness makes sense for everyone, including fire and emergency service personnel, the taxpayers, and the public served.

National Fire Protection Association Standards

In 2008, the NFPA released NFPA 1583, *Standard on Health-Related Fitness Programs for Fire Department Members*. As the NFPA states, "The purpose of this standard is to provide the minimum requirements for a health-related fitness program for fire department members that enhances the members' ability to perform occupational activities efficiently and safely and reduces the risk of injury, disease, and premature death.

"The health-related fitness program shall include the following components:

Assignment of a qualified health and fitness coordinator
Periodic fitness assessment for all members
Exercise training program that is available to all members
Education and counseling regarding health promotion for all members
Process for collecting and maintaining health-related fitness program data"[17]

When adopted, this standard can be a key component of any occupational safety and health program, and is a companion to NFPA 1582, *Comprehensive Occupational Medical Program for Fire Departments,* 2007 Edition.

Reprinted with permission from the NFPA 1583-2008: *Standard on Health-Related Fitness Programs for Fire Department Members*© 2008, National Fire Protection Association, Quincy, MA. This reprinted material is not the complete and official position of the NFPA on the referenced subject, which is represented only by the standard in its entirety.

National Volunteer Fire Council Heart-Healthy Firefighter Program

Each year, heart attack is the leading cause of line-of-duty deaths for firefighters. In a proactive effort to reduce the number of firefighters dying from heart disease and keep the Nation's first responders healthy, the NVFC launched the Heart-Healthy Firefighter Program in 2003 to promote fitness, nutrition, and health awareness within America's fire and emergency services. It is the Nation's only heart attack prevention and awareness campaign targeted at all firefighters and EMS personnel, both volunteer and career.

As part of the program, the NVFC provides tools and resources to assist firefighters, EMS personnel, and their families in becoming and staying heart-healthy. More information about each of these resources is available on the Heart-Healthy Firefighter Web site at **www.healthy-firefighter.org** Some of the tools and resources are

- *Trade Show Booth.* The NVFC brings its interactive booth to emergency service trade shows across the country. The NVFC has partnered with L&T Health and Fitness, an award-winning fitness management and health promotion company, to provide free health screenings to firefighters, EMS personnel, and their families. By the end of 2007, over 14,000 first responders had been screened for heart disease risk factors including blood pressure, cholesterol, and body composition. The booth also features cooking demonstrations to show attendees that heart-healthy cooking can be easy and taste great.

- *Web Site.* The Heart-Healthy Firefighter Program Web site at **www.healthy-firefighter.org** contains resources to help first responders, their departments, and their families on the road to heart health. The Web site offers information on heart basics, fitness, nutrition, and lifestyle choices, as well as customized features such as "Tools for Firefighters" and "Tools for Families." The site also contains tools to help implement and maintain a heart-healthy lifestyle including the Fired Up For Fitness Challenge, heart-healthy recipes, and motivational firefighter success stories.

- *Fitness Challenge.* The Fired Up For Fitness Challenge is an interactive program where firefighters and EMS personnel can design and implement their individual fitness program. Participants measure personal progress by recording their physical activity and results such as weight loss, as well as compare their progress with fellow first responders across the Nation. Participants also qualify for rewards as they reach certain benchmarks.

- *Cookbook. The Heart-Healthy Firefighter Cookbook* includes over 60 delicious yet healthy recipes that firefighters and EMS personnel can use either at home or at the station. Many of the recipes were submitted by firefighters who already have committed to becoming heart-healthy.

- *Resource Guide. The Heart-Healthy Firefighter Resource Guide* is available both in print form and for free download on the Heart-Healthy Firefighter Web site. The Guide contains all the information needed to start on the path to a heart-healthy lifestyle. Sections cover essential heart-health information, risk factors, and lifestyle choices.

- *Newsletter. The Pulse* is a printed, quarterly newsletter that includes ideas, resources, advice, and information to keep firefighters and EMS personnel healthy throughout the year. Readers also can contribute by submitting success stories about becoming heart healthy, ideas or suggestions about aspects of maintaining a heart-healthy lifestyle, or questions about the program or heart health.

- *E-news.* The Heart-Healthy Firefighter E-news is a monthly electronic newsletter that contains program and health news, tips for a heart-healthy lifestyle, upcoming events, and more.

In addition, the NVFC is developing two new components that will bring the Heart-Healthy Firefighter Program to the department level. The first is a Health and Fitness Advocate Program, designed to train fire and emergency services personnel on how to create and maintain an effective health and wellness program within their department, with a significant focus on heart-health. The second new component is the Adopt the Program initiative that allows firefighters and departments to register with the Heart-Healthy Firefighter Program to receive specific tools and information that they can follow to maintain a heart-healthy lifestyle. These include meal plans, fitness information, and tracking mechanisms to monitor progress.

International Association of Fire Fighters/International Association of Fire Chiefs Wellness-Fitness Initiative

The International Association of Firefighters/International Association of Fire Chiefs (IAFF/IAFC) Joint Labor Management Wellness-Fitness Initiative (WFI) is an unprecedented endeavor to join together labor and management to evaluate and improve the health, wellness, and fitness of firefighters and emergency medical services (EMS) providers.

Ten U.S. cities and Canadian career fire departments participate in the WFI Task Force, which was first convened in 1996. The participating departments and their IAFF local affiliate have all formally committed to adopt the WFI and to continue participation in the program. A key aspect of the program is that it be implemented in full, not just selected components, although it is acceptable to implement one or two components at a time until full implementation is achieved. Although developed by career departments, the WFI can be implemented in career, combination, or volunteer departments.

The WFI is based on the premise that the program is mandatory, nonpunitive, and confidential. If a volunteer firefighter wellness program is to succeed, these same conditions should apply. According to the WFI manual, "all component results are measured against the individual's previous examination and assessments and not against any standard or norm." Confidentiality of medical information is the most critical aspect of the WFI. The unauthorized release of personal details which may be recorded as part of a medical evaluation causes legal, ethical, and personal problems for the employee, employer, and examining physician. All information obtained from medical and physical evaluations must be considered confidential, and the employer will only have access to information regarding fitness for duty, necessary work restrictions, and if needed, appropriate accommodations. Also, all medical information must be maintained in separate files from all other personnel information.

The 10 U.S. fire departments participating in the program are

- Austin Fire Department (Texas);
- Calgary Fire Department (Canada);
- Charlotte Fire Department (North Carolina);
- Fairfax County Fire and Rescue Department (Virginia);
- Indianapolis Fire Department (Indiana);
- Los Angeles Fire Department (California);
- Miami-Dade Fire Rescue Department (Florida);
- City of New York Fire Department (New York);

- Phoenix Fire Department (Arizona); and
- Seattle Fire Department (Washington).

Table 2. Components of the International Association of Fire Fighters - International Association of Fire Chiefs Initiative.

Category	COMPONENTS
MEDICAL	• Physical Evaluation • Body Composition Evaluation • Laboratory Tests • Vision Tests • Hearing Evaluations • Spirometry • Electrocardiogram • Cancer Screening • Immunizations and Infectious Disease Testing • Referrals • Data Collection
FITNESS	• Medical Clearance • Onduty Time for Exercise • Equipment and Facilities • Exercise Specialists and Peer Trainers • Fitness Incorporated into Philosophy • Fitness Evaluations (aerobic capabilities, flexibility, muscular strength, muscular endurance) • Fitness Self-Assessments • Exercise Prescriptions
REHABILITATION	• Need for Rehabilitation • Rehabilitation as a Priority • Establishment of a Medical Liaison • Physical Therapy Services • Clinical Pathways • Alternate Duty • Injury Prevention Program
BEHAVIORAL HEALTH	• Professional Assistance • Nutrition • Tobacco Use Cessation • Employee Assistance Programs • Substance Abuse Intervention • Stress Management • Critical Incident Stress Management • Chaplain Services

All 10 of the departments have implemented the program to some degree, and numerous other departments have implemented the program as well. The third Edition of the WFI was released in August of 2008.

Components of the Wellness-Fitness Initiative. As seen in Table 2, the WFI has multiple components, all of which are designed to be implemented as a whole. In the case of the volunteer service, it would be quite challenging to implement all of these components at once. Many of the components are discussed in further detail in the chapter on developing a model program, later in this guide. In addition to the information provided in Table 2, the third edition of the WFI now contains chapters on cost justification, demonstrating the cost/benefits of implementing the WFI, and an implementation chapter that includes additional resources designed to assist the department in setting up the WFI.

Candidate Physical Ability Test (CPAT). This program was developed as a fair and valid evaluation tool to assist in the selection of firefighters, and to ensure that all firefighter candidates possess the physical ability to complete critical tasks effectively and safely. The CPAT Program covers every aspect of administering the CPAT, including recruiting and mentoring programs, providing recruits with fitness guidance to help prepare them for the CPAT, and setting up and administering the test. In our ongoing effort to ensure that the CPAT is being used properly and only as intended, the IAFF has enacted a formal licensing policy that will affect the way in which this program can be used legally.

Peer Fitness Trainers. The IAFF/IAFC Wellness-Fitness Task Force has determined that successful implementation of the Wellness-Fitness Initiative and the CPAT programs require a trained firefighter in each department who can take the lead. These individuals must have the ability to design and implement fitness programs, to improve the wellness and fitness of his or her department, to assist with the physical training of recruits, and assist the broader community in achieving wellness and fitness (e.g., fitness programs in schools). This need for a department-level leader led to the development of the Fire Service Peer Fitness Trainer (PFT) certification program. The PFT certification is provided and sponsored by the IAFF/IAFC with the American Council on Exercise (ACE).

This certification provides fire department personnel with the knowledge needed to develop exercise programs for other department personnel. PFTs also learn WFI testing protocols, how to proctor the CPAT, and are helpful in promoting wellness and fitness throughout their departments. Since the program's inception in 2004, 144 workshops in 34 States, Washington, DC, and three

Canadian provinces have been conducted with over 4,200 firefighters participating in the certification classes and sitting for the certification exam. For more information on the PFT course, visit **http://www.iaff.org/HS/PFT/ peer_%20index.htm**

U.S. Air Force Physical Fitness Program

The U.S. Air Force Fitness Program was launched on January 1, 2004. This program replaces the annual ergo-cycle test that the Air Force had previously used for several years. The following requirements are for after basic training and technical school. Recruits in basic training and non-prior-service recruits in technical school continue to be tested using basic training standards.

Under the U.S. Air Force Fitness Program, fitness points are awarded in four areas: aerobic (running), body composition, pushups, and crunches. Those who are not medically cleared to run take the ergo-cycle test for the aerobic portion. Ratings are Excellent (90 or above), Good (75 to 89.9), and Fail (below 75). Individuals who fail must be re-tested within 90 days. In 2007, the Air Force announced that fitness test results (pass/fail) will be included on all future performance reports, so failing the fitness test can have a significant negative impact on an Air Force member's career (promotions, assignments, retention, etc.).

Members must complete all components unless medically exempted. If medically exempted from any component, the total score is calculated as the total component points achieved times 100, divided by the total number of possible points. The maximum component points are: aerobic (50), body composition (30), pushups (10), and crunches (10). Results are then compared to male and female fitness component charts.[18]

End Notes

[1] United States Fire Administration, *Firefighter Fatalities in the United States in 2006.*

[2] Ibid.

[3] United States Fire Administration Fallen Firefighters Memorial Database Online. http://www. usfa.fema.gov/applications/ffmem/ffmem_search.cfm?p_mn_status=1&p_death_year=2007 Accessed February 28, 2008.

[4] Karter, Michael, and Joseph Molis, Op. cit.

[5] Hall, John, et al. *Four Years Later–A Second Needs Assessment of the U.S. Fire Service.* NFPA/FEMA/USFA, Oct. 2006.

[6] USFA, *Firefighter Fatalities.*

[7] Ibid.

[8] Reuters Health, July 17, 2001.

[9] United States Fire Administration. *Fire-Related Firefighter Injuries in 2004*. Feb. 2008.

[10] Karter, Michael. *Patterns of Firefighter Fireground Injuries*. National Fire Protection Association, 2007.

[11] United States Fire Administration. *Fire and Emergency Medical Services Ergonomics–A Guide for Understanding and Implementing An Ergonomics Program in Your Department*. Mar. 1996.

[12] Stewart, Gord. "Fire Fitness – Coping with Life on the Job."
http://www.cfpsa.com/en/psp/fitness/fire_fitness/coping.asp (Accessed August 15, 2003)

[13] Wright, Brad. "Surgeon General to Cops: Put Down the Donuts." March 2, 2003.
http://www.cnn.com/2003/HEALTH/02/28/obesity.police/ (Accessed July 25, 2003)

[14] Thompson, Jamie. "Lifestyle: Making the Right Choices." August 17, 2007.
http://www.firerescue1.com/health/articles/293034 (Accessed June 12, 2008)

[15] Kay, Bridget, et al. "Assessment of Firefighter's Cardiovascular Disease-Related Knowledge and Behaviors." *Journal of American Dietetic Association*. Vol. 101, No. 7, July 2001.

[16] Stefano, Michael (adapted from). "Avoid 5 Reasons Fitness Plans Fail."
www.howtobefit.com/fitness-success-plan.htm

[17] Reprinted with permission from NFPA 1583-2008, *Standard on Health-Related Fitness Programs for Fire Department Members*. Copyright© 2008, National Fire Protection, Quincy, MA. This reprinted material is not the complete and official position of the NFPA on the referenced subject, which is represented only by the standard in its entirety.

[18] Powers, Rod (adapted from). "Air Force Fitness Test." 2007.
http://usmilitary.about.com/od/airforce/a/affitness.htm (Accessed February 1, 2008)

In: Firefighter Fitness: A Health and Wellness Guide   ISBN: 978-1-60741-650-0
Editor: Ernest L. Schneider   © 2010 Nova Science Publishers, Inc.

Chapter 3

IMPORTANCE OF HEALTH AND WELLNESS IN THE VOLUNTEER FIRE AND EMERGENCY SERVICES

U.S. Fire Administration

Chapter II looked at the state of health and wellness in the volunteer fire and emergency services. As the statistics showed, heart attacks represent the leading cause of onduty death, while sprains and strains represent the number-one cause of injuries. This chapter will look at why it is important for volunteer firefighters and emergency medical personnel to reduce their risk of these health issues.

CARDIOVASCULAR DISEASE

Cardiovascular disease (CVD) is the leading cause of death in the United States, accounting for approximately 650,000 deaths per year.[1] It exacts a considerable toll on the fire service, as shown in the previous chapter.

USFA and the NVFC aim to reduce drastically the number of firefighter deaths due to heart attacks. A commitment to health and safety requires that the fire and emergency services continue to address line-of-duty deaths due to other causes through proper training, adequate resources, etc. This Guide, however, is aimed at improving first responder health and safety by addressing the important health issue of CVD in the fire and emergency services. This chapter outlines the development of CVD, the risk factors for developing it, the relative risk associated with different values for each risk factor, and the benefits of exercise in controlling risk factors.

CVD refers collectively to a state of disease in the blood vessels. If blood vessels become narrowed (i.e., by the buildup of plaque) or obstructed (i.e., by a blood clot), then blood and the oxygen and nutrients it carries, cannot be delivered to the vital organs of the body. If blood flow to the heart muscle is impeded, a heart attack occurs. The terms coronary heart disease (CHD) or coronary artery disease (CAD) describe a specific form of CVD in which the blood vessels supplying the heart muscle are blocked.

When there is an obstruction in a coronary vessel, the tissue below the blockage does not get adequate oxygen. If the lack of oxygen (called ischemia) is too severe, the heart tissue dies (called an infarction; a myocardial infarction means death of heart muscle tissue). Thus, a person who has suffered a myocardial infarction (also called a heart attack) has had a portion of the heart tissue destroyed. If the area supplied by the blood vessel is very small, the person may recover from the heart attack or may not even know that he or she has suffered a heart attack. However, if the area below the occlusion is too great, the heart cannot continue to function as an effective pump, and death results.

Atherosclerosis refers to the disease condition in which plaque builds up in the arterial wall causing the size of the vessel opening to become narrower. The initiation of atherosclerotic plaque buildup may begin quite early in life. In fact, there is strong evidence that it begins in the early 20s for many people in developed countries of the Western world. Therefore, it is important to think of CVD as a long-term disease that begins early in life, although symptoms are often delayed until middle or older age. Also, CVD can reach advanced stages without overt symptoms. In many individuals, the first sign of CVD is a fatal heart attack, thus reinforcing the need for young first responders to take steps to avoid or delay atherosclerosis. It also suggests that all firefighters and EMS personnel should seriously address the health issues of CVD, even if they are symptom-free.

A health risk factor is a characteristic that is present early in life and is associated with an increased risk of developing future disease. A modifiable risk factor is a risk factor that can be minimized by diet, exercise, or personal habits. There are several risk factors for CVD, including nonmodifiable and modifiable ones (see Table 3). The nonmodifiable risk factors include gender, age, race, and family history. Men are more likely to suffer CVD at a younger age than females; thus, being over 45 years is considered a risk factor for males, and being over 55 years is a risk factor for females. Family history is defined as the premature death (before 55 years for males or before 65 years for females) of a parent or sibling from CVD.

Modifiable risk factors deserve a great deal of attention because, when they are altered, an individual can influence his or her likelihood of developing CVD. There are six major modifiable risk factors: smoking, hypertension (high blood pressure), hypercholesterolemia (high cholesterol levels), diabetes or impaired glucose tolerance, obesity, and physical activity. The more risk factors that an individual has, the greater the likelihood he or she will suffer from CVD.

Table 3. Risk Factors for Developing Cardiovascular Disease

Risk Factors That Cannot be Modified	Risk Factors That Can be Modified
• Age • Heredity • Race • Gender	• Cholesterol-lipid fractions • Cigarette smoking • Diabetes mellitus • Hypertension • Obesity • Physical inactivity

Smoking

Approximately 21 percent of the adult population in the United States smoke, and approximately 4,000 young people begin to smoke each day.[2] Cigarette smoking accounts for an estimated 438,000 deaths per year in the United States, more than 20 percent of them due to cardiovascular disease.[3] In fact, as early as 1983, the Surgeon General established smoking as the leading avoidable cause of CVD. Thus, quitting cigarette smoking is one of the most important interventions possible to decrease the risk of premature death due to CVD. Smoking increases the risk for sudden cardiac death, aortic aneurysm, peripheral vascular disease, and stroke. Smoking one pack of cigarettes per day doubles the risk of CVD compared to not smoking.[4] As the number of cigarettes smoked increases, so does the risk of coronary artery disease and stroke.

Hypertension

Hypertension refers to a chronic, persistent elevation of blood pressure. Epidemiological data shows that the risk of death doubles with a systolic blood pressure greater than or equal to 140 mmHg and a diastolic blood pressure greater than or equal to 90, and thus a blood pressure above 140/90 is defined as hypertension. The risk of developing CVD increases directly with increasing levels of both systolic and diastolic blood pressure. Untreated hypertension can lead to stroke, heart attack, heart failure, and kidney damage.[5]

The primary lifestyle modifications to help reduce hypertension include smoking cessation, diet and exercise, with the overall goals of losing weight, increasing physical activity levels, and decreasing salt intake. A program of regular aerobic exercise results in a decrease of approximately 10 mmHg in systolic and diastolic blood pressure in hypertensive individuals.[6] Exercise also helps control blood glucose levels and the ability of blood vessels to change diameter during exercise.

High Cholesterol

Blood lipids are comprised primarily of triglycerides and cholesterol. Cholesterol and triglycerides are carried in the blood by a lipoprotein molecule. Low-density lipoproteins (LDLs), also known as "bad cholesterol", and high-density lipoproteins (HDLs), also known as "good cholesterol", vary in their densities and in the way they transport cholesterol. Elevated levels of triglycerides, cholesterol, and LDL-cholesterol are associated with increased risk of CVD. On the other hand, increased levels of HDL-cholesterol are associated with a decreased risk of CVD. Therefore, elevated levels of HDL are desirable— they actually help decrease the risk of CVD.

Elevated levels of cholesterol in young adults greatly increase their risk of CHD later in life. In fact, young men who are in the upper quartile (highest 25 percent for cholesterol levels) have a nine-fold increase in risk of heart attack compared to men in the lowest quartile (lowest 25 percent).[7] The risk of CVD increases progressively with increasing levels of cholesterol; there is a 20- to 30-percent increase in risk for CHD for every 10 mg/dl increase in cholesterol.[8] Exercise is an important component of any weight loss program and weight loss is associated with positive changes in lipid profiles. Furthermore, regular aerobic exercise decreases triglyceride levels and increases HDL levels.

Obesity

Despite what seems to be an obsession with thinness and dieting, approximately 33 percent of the adult population in the United States is obese, and another 30 to 35 percent of the population is overweight.[9] Obesity is associated with a number of diseases, including CVD (high blood pressure, dyslipidemia (altered or dysfunctional levels of lipids in the blood)), diabetes, gallbladder disease, and cancer. Obesity is associated with several other risk factors but it does appear that it also exerts an independent influence on the risk of CVD.

As excess body weight increases so does the risk of CVD.[10] There is little or no change in mortality at the lower end of the range (Body Mass Index (BMI) less than 25), but as BMI increases above 25, risk increases substantially. Thus, each incremental pound gained (once a person is categorized as overweight) is associated with additional risk.

Studies have consistently shown that exercise is particularly effective in maintaining weight loss. Additionally, exercise is the best way to lose fat and maintain muscle mass. When a person loses weight through diet alone, he/she loses fat and muscle. On the other hand, a person who loses weight through a combination of diet and exercise loses fat weight almost exclusively.

Diabetes

Diabetes is a metabolic disorder characterized by the inability to use sugar (glucose) effectively. Individuals with diabetes have a 300 percent to 500 percent increased risk of cardiac events. According to the American Diabetes Association, 65 percent of all deaths among diabetic patients are from heart disease or stroke.[11]

The degree of cardiovascular risk is directly related to fasting blood glucose levels.[12] Additionally, individuals who have diabetes along with other risk factors are at much higher risk than nondiabetic individuals with the same number of risk factors. Diabetes often coexists with other risk factors for CVD. In fact, the cluster of risk factors has been termed metabolic syndrome X, and includes abdominal obesity, hypertension, dyslipidemia, and an inability to effectively use glucose (diabetes). Therefore, it is important that persons with diabetes very aggressively control other risk factors; they should lose excess body weight, exercise regularly, and eat a diet low in simple sugars and carbohydrates.

Physical Inactivity

Physical inactivity is related to several of the risk factors discussed previously. A lack of exercise increases an individual's risk of obesity, hypertension, dyslipidemia, and diabetes. However, physical inactivity is also an independent risk factor for CVD. The risk of CVD in inactive people is about twice that of physically active individuals; approximately the same as for hypertension and high cholesterol.[13] In fact, physical inactivity is responsible for approximately 200,000 deaths per year in the United States.[14] Numerous studies have shown that CVD mortality is inversely related to level of physical activity or fitness.[15]

Summary

CVD is a major threat to the health and safety of firefighters and EMS personnel. To stay healthy and address the risk factors for developing CVD, first responders should adopt a few healthy lifestyle habits. In short, to reduce the risk of suffering a heart attack or stroke, it is imperative that firefighters:

- do not smoke;
- follow a regimen of moderate aerobic exercise; and
- eat a balanced diet, avoiding excess saturated fats, excess simple sugars, and maintaining normal body weight.

Table 4 details the recommendations above and indicates the risk factors that are influenced by each recommendation. Of particular note is the benefit physical activity has on five of the six modifiable risk factors. Imagine the excitement within the fire and emergency services, indeed the Nation, if a medication were developed that could achieve half the benefits that we know can be derived from consistent participation in a moderate exercise program!

Table 4. Recommendations for Decreasing CVD Risk Factors

Recommendations	Risk Factor Influenced
Exercise Moderately	• Decreased blood pressure • Improved lipid (cholesterol) profile • Decreased body fat • Improved glucose tolerance • Eliminates physical inactivity
Eat a Balanced Diet	• Improved lipid (cholesterol) profile • Decreased body weight • Improved glucose tolerance • May decrease blood pressure
Do not Smoke	• Decreased artery blockage • Increased lung health capacity

IMPORTANCE OF IMPROVED STRENGTH AND FLEXIBILITY

Strength and flexibility training can effectively develop musculoskeletal strength, musculoskeletal endurance, and functional movement around the joints, and is strongly recommended for health, fitness, injury prevention, rehabilitation, and for improving one's overall quality of life.

Flexibility is the ability to move a joint freely through an entire range of motion. As an example, good shoulder flexibility should allow both hands to touch together behind your back. It is, however, joint-specific, varying significantly across joints and between individuals. Many factors including joint structure, ligaments, tendons, muscles, skin, fat tissue, body temperature, gender, and age all contribute to the range of motion at a joint.[16]

Many muscular and skeletal problems result from poor flexibility. For adults, this is typically the most neglected aspect of a physical fitness program. Most individuals can benefit from improved flexibility, regardless of age or gender. With aging, muscles shorten (tighten), diminishing the range of motion in a joint, hindering or halting day-to-day activities and movements. A regular stretching program can help lengthen your muscles, and maintain or restore flexibility.

The benefits of being flexible include

- **Flexibility decreases risk of injury.** Increasing range of motion decreases the resistance in various tissues. An individual is therefore less likely to incur injury by exceeding tissue extensibility, or maximum range of movement of tissues during activity.[17]

- **Flexibility increases physical efficiency and performance.** A flexible joint has the ability to move farther in its range and requires less energy to do so.[18]

- **Flexibility increases tissue temperature.** An increase in tissue temperature increases circulation and nutrient transport due to decreased joint viscosity.[19]

- **Flexibility increases neuromuscular coordination.** An increase in coordination, or ease of movement, occurs because of an increase in nerve impulse velocity. In attuning the central nervous system to the physical demands placed upon it, opposing muscle groups work in a more synergistic or coordinated fashion.[20]

- **Flexibility training reduces muscle soreness.** Postexercise stretching is extremely effective in reducing localized, muscular soreness, typically experienced 12 to 72 hours after exercise.[21]

The American College of Sports Medicine, American Heart Association (AHA), Centers for Disease Control and Prevention (CDC), and the U.S. Surgeon General's Office consider strength training to be an integral part of any comprehensive health program and have defined population-specific guidelines.[22, 23] The benefits of a strength training program include

- **Improved body composition, muscle growth, and metabolism.** Effectively designed strength training programs stimulate muscle growth, burning additional calories and lowering the amount of fat on the body. All individuals of any age or gender can build muscle effectively. A 1-pound increase in muscle mass can increase caloric expenditure by 30 to 50 calories per day. Muscle losses attributed to injury, aging, or inactivity can reduce your caloric expenditure by the same amount.[24]
- **Improved physical functioning.** The neuromuscular adaptations to strength training enable one to perform tasks with less physiological stress. Much of the improved efficiency demonstrated with strength

training is attributed to neural and hormonal adaptations that increase neural drive to muscles; improve muscle recruitment and synchronization; increase muscle contractile activation; and diminish the protective function of proprioceptors that limit range, intensity, and speed of movements around joints.[25]

- **Decreased risk for osteoporosis and osteoarthritis.** Weight training will increase bone density, which is of great concern as we age or become postmenopausal. Increased bone density reduces the chances of bone fractures and bone degeneration. Additionally, strengthening joints and muscles supporting the joints can reduce joint pain and inflammation significantly.

- **Improved flexibility.** Optimal musculoskeletal function maintains adequate range of motion in all joints. This is of particular importance to the lower back region, where lack of flexibility from insufficient activity or poor posture increases the risk of chronic low back pain.

ERGONOMIC-RELATED DISORDERS

This section has been adapted from the USFA guide: *Fire and Emergency Medical Services Ergonomics–A Guide for Understanding and Implementing An Ergonomics Program in Your Department.*[26] This guide is considered to be the foremost authority on ergonomic issues in the fire and emergency services.

Ergonomic-related disorders include cumulative trauma disorders and back disorders. Alone, these injuries, which often are developed over time as a result of uncorrected behaviors, postures, and habits, pose threats. When combined with the rough nature of the fireground, with its requirements of increased physicality, strength, and agility, ergonomic-related disorders can increase the risk for prolonged injury and can risk first responder lives if untreated.

Often, ergonomic-related disorders may appear minor, but such disorders can exacerbate fireground sprains and strains severely and transform moderate injuries into more threatening injuries that increase job time lost, and diminish both dexterity and the ability to fight fires effectively. The ergonomic-related disorders discussed in this section often are preventable and treatable through a fitness program, behavioral modification program, and screenings and assessments. Understanding the disorders themselves, their risks, and their causes is critical to the design of an effective health and wellness program.

Cumulative Trauma Disorders

CTDs can be described as wear and tear on joints and surrounding tissue because of overuse. Potentially, every joint in the body can be affected, but the joints in the lower back and upper limbs receive the most injuries. Cumulative disorders accumulate through time. Acute trauma, by contrast, is injuries that occur as the result of a onetime event, such as a cut or fall. Cumulative trauma is known by a variety of terms, such as musculoskeletal disorders, overuse syndrome, or repetitive motion disorders.

CTDs affect any area of the body where tendons, joints, and nerves are found. Most commonly, CTDs target the upper extremities, which include all of the anatomical components from the shoulder to the fingers. While acute injuries resulting from a single event do occur to the upper extremity, more disorders are currently recognized as the cumulative effect of multiple small, often unrecognized, repetitive injuries, particularly those for the back. Upper extremity CTDs largely affect the origin of muscles (where the muscle attaches to the bone, the tendon, the joints, the blood vessels, and the nerves).

Types of Cumulative Trauma Disorders

While there are several types of CTDs, most CTDs fall into two main categories:

Tendonitis. Tendons serve as links that connect muscle to bone and come into play whenever a muscle is used for the motion of a bone structure. In some areas of the body, tendons slide through sheaths. As with any other moving part, overuse of tendons can cause friction, which in turn causes wear and tear and expansion or swelling. When tendons or their sheaths swell, there is pain and tenderness, known as tendonitis.

Nerve compression. Nerves are found throughout the body and several points exist where it is possible for nerves to be compressed. Pinching of nerves is often caused by making certain awkward motions or assuming certain postures. Other times, compression can be caused by swelling of nearby tendons.

Risk Factors

Several on-the-job factors can increase the risk of developing CTDs. The more factors involved and the greater the exposure to each, the higher the chance of developing a disorder. Factors of working conditions include

- *Repetition.* Risk increases with number and frequency of motions made by a particular part of the body.

- *Force.* Risk increases with the amount of exertion required for particular motions.

- *Awkward postures.* Risk increases with positions of the body, which deviate from a neutral position; primarily bent wrists, elbows away from their normal positions at the side of the body, and a bent or twisted lower back.

- *Contact stress.* Risk increases with excessive contact between sensitive body tissue and sharp edges or unforgiving surfaces on a tool or piece of equipment.

- *Vibration.* Risk increases with exposure to vibrating tools or equipment, whether a hand-held power tool or whole-body vibration.

- *Temperature extremes.* Risk increases with exposure to excessive heat or cold.

- *Stressful conditions.* Risk increases with certain stressful situations at work or due to the nature of the work.

Back Disorders

The back is a complex system consisting of several distinct spinal regions. Lifting, bending, and twisting motions (on or off the job) can cause severe injury and pain. Next to the common cold, back disorder is the reason most often cited for job absenteeism.

Types of Disorders

Pulled or strained muscles, ligaments, tendons, and discs are perhaps the most common back problems. Half of the U.S. workforce is likely to experience back problems at least once during a lifetime. Most back disorders result from chronic, or long-term, injury rather than from one specific incident. When back muscles or ligaments are injured from repetitive pulling and straining, the back muscles, discs, and ligaments can become scarred and weakened and lose their ability to support the back. This condition makes additional injuries more likely. Types of back disorders include

- *Lumbosacral strain.* Caused by overuse of the muscles of the lumbar and sacral areas of the back.

- *Sacroiliitis.* Caused by inflammation from overuse of the lumbar muscles of the joints between the lowest and sacral areas of the back, spinal bones (sacrum), and the hip bones (ilium).

- *Lumbosacral sprain.* Caused by overuse of ligaments in the lumbar and sacral areas of the back.

- *Postural low back pain.* Results from overuse of the lumbosacral muscles by maintaining a posture that requires these muscles to work beyond their capabilities.

- *Muscular insufficiency.* Occurs when muscles are unable to bear stresses imposed on them.

- *Herniated disc.* Results when the disc that sits between two spinal bones (vertebrae) bulges from between them.

- *Degenerated disc.* Results when wear and tear on disc slowly destroys its structure.

Risk Factors

Back disorders frequently are caused by the cumulative effects of faulty body mechanics such as excessive twisting, bending, reaching, lifting loads that are too heavy, too big, or too far from the body, staying in one position for too long, poor physical conditions, and poor posture. Prolonged sitting stresses the body, particularly the lower back and the thighs. It may cause the lower back to bow outward if there is inadequate support. This abnormal curvature can lead to painful lower back problems, a common complaint among office workers. Other risk factors include

- *Heavy physical work.* Information based on workers' compensation claims and insurance data show that low-back pain is more prevalent in highly physical jobs where the potential for overexertion injuries is greater.

- **Lifting.** Low-back pain is clearly triggered by lifting; the weight, speed, duration, and frequency of lifting affect the onset of low-back pain.

- **Bending, stretching, and reaching.** Bending in combination with lifting appears to be the most common cause for low-back pain; the incident of low-back pain also increases with loads held away from the body.

- **Twisting.** Lifting in combination with twisting has been implicated in low-back pain injuries.

- **Pushing and pulling.** Pulling and pushing account for 9 to 18 percent of all back strains and sprains.

- **Prolonged sitting and standing.** Studies show that jobs involving all standing or all sitting postures are associated with increased risk for low-back pain as compared to jobs involving frequent changes in posture.

- **Vibrations.** As in other CTDs, vibration is a significant risk factor.

- **Accidents.** Traumatic events outside the context of manual lifting, such as slipping, tripping, stumbling, or other incidents, which place unexpected loads on the back, can contribute to chronic low-back pain.

Between complications of CVD, strains, sprains, and other ergonomic-related disorders, firefighting is truly one of the most dangerous occupations. The demands of firefighters are very high and require a focus on health and wellness. This chapter looked at some of the health risks of the emergency services.

End Notes

[1] Heron, Melonie P., et al. "Deaths: Final Data for 2004." *National Vital Statistics Reports,* Vol. 55 #19, 2007.

[2] Centers for Disease Control and Prevention. *Annual Smoking-Attributable Mortality, Years of Potential Life Lost, and Productivity Losses–United States, 1997–2001.* Morbidity and Mortality Weekly Report [serial online]. 2002;51(14):300–303 [cited 2006 Dec 5]. Available from: http://www.cdc.gov/mmwr/preview/mmwrhtml/mm5114a2.htm

[3] Ibid.

[4] Ridker, P.M., J. Genest, Jr., and P. Libby. "Risk Factors for Atherosclerotic Disease." In: Braumwald, E., Zipes, D.P., and Libby, P. (eds). *Heart Disease: A Textbook of Cardiovascular Medicine*. 6th Ed. Philadelphia: W.B. Saunders, 2001.

[5] Plowman, S.A., and Denise Smith, *Exercise Physiology: for Health, Fitness, and Performance*. San Francisco: Benjamin Cummings, 2003.

[6] Ibid.

[7] Oberman, A. "Role of Lipids in the Prevention of Cardiovascular Disease." *Clinical Reviews*, 10-15, Spring 2000.

[8] Gaziano, J.M., J.E. Mason, and P.M. Ridker. "Primary and Secondary Prevention of Coronary Heart Disease." In: Braumwald, E., D.P. Zipes, and P. Libby, (eds). *Heart Disease: A Textbook of Cardiovascular Medicine*. 6th Ed. Philadelphia: W.B. Saunders, 2001.

[9] Ogden C.L., Carroll M.D., Curtin L.R., McDowell M.A., Tabak C.J., and Flegal K.M. "Prevalence of Overweight and Obesity in the United States, 1999-2004." JAMA 295:1549-1555, 2006.

[10] Manson, et al. "A Prospective Study of Obesity and Risk of Coronary Heart Disease in Women." *New England Journal of Medicine,* 322:882-889, 1990.

[11] American Diabetes Association. "Diabetes and Cardiovascular (Heart) Disease." www.diabetes.org/diabetes-statistics/heart-disease.jsp (Accessed July 2008).

[12] Nesto, R.W., and L. Libby. In: Braumwald, Zipes, and Libby. *Heart Disease: A Textbook of Cardiovascular Medicine*. 6th Ed. Philadelphia: W.B. Saunders, 2001. ·   · ··

[13] Plowman and Smith, Op. cit.

[14] Ridker, Genest, and Libby, Op. cit.

[15] Haskell, W.S.L. "Health Consequences of Physical Activity: Understanding and Challenges Regarding Dose Response." *Medicine and Science in Sports and Exercise,* 26(6):649-660, 1994.

[16] American College of Sports Medicine (ACSM). *Resource Manual for Guidelines for Exercise Testing and Prescription,* 4th Ed. Baltimore: Lippincott, Williams & Wilkins, 2001.

[17] National Strength and Conditioning Association. Essentials of Strength Training and Conditioning. 2nd Ed. Champaign: Human Kinetics, 2000.

[18] ACSM, Op. cit.

[19] Ibid.

[20] National Strength and Conditioning Association, Op. cit.

[21] ACSM, Op. cit.

[22] Ibid.

[23] United States Department of Health and Human Services "Physical Activity and Health: A Report of the Surgeon General." Atlanta: Centers for Disease Control and Prevention, National Center for Chronic Disease Prevention and Health Promotion, 1996.

[24] ACSM, Op. cit.

[25] Fleck S.J., et al. "Designing Resistance Training Programs." Champaign: Human Kinetics, 1987.

[26] United States Fire Administration. *Fire and Emergency Medical Services Ergonomics–A Guide for Understanding and Implementing An Ergonomics Program in Your Department.*

In: Firefighter Fitness: A Health and Wellness Guide   ISBN: 978-1-60741-650-0
Editor: Ernest L. Schneider   © 2010 Nova Science Publishers, Inc.

Chapter 4

VOLUNTEER PROGRAMS FROM ACROSS THE NATION

U.S. Fire Administration

Previous chapters of this Guide have addressed why it is important for volunteers and the departments they serve to focus on health and wellness. This chapter looks at programs implemented by various volunteer or combination fire and emergency service departments across the country to assess the strengths and weaknesses of each program. This assessment, or "lessons learned," is a valuable tool for departments that want to implement their own programs.

OVERVIEW OF CURRENT HEALTH AND WELLNESS PROGRAMS

In 2003, the NVFC State directors identified 16 volunteer departments with current experience with health and wellness programs. The departments varied widely in type, membership size, and community served.

Most of the programs studied began in the early 1990s and, with one exception, remained viable. Less than half of the departments reported a positive reception to the program, and 63 percent noted fire service culture as an impediment to the program. Participation was spread evenly among age groups, but a smaller percentage of women participated than men. The three greatest problem areas with the programs were

- lack of funding;
- lack of well-defined requirements; and
- inability to keep membership motivated.

The departments used many different approaches to health and wellness including screenings, examinations, immunizations, education, behavioral modifications, and fitness programming. Fifty-six percent of the departments analyzed injury reports to customize the health and wellness program to meet the needs of their department.

Most departments acknowledged that, while the time and equipment are available for programming, active participation by the members was quite low. For example, 56 percent of the departments offered training and educational components to improve mental and physical health and quality of life, but the use was only sporadic.

Seventy-five percent of the departments ensured immunizations for Hepatitis B and Tetanus, and provided annual flu shots. Sixty-three percent provided full blood laboratory screening and full medical physical examinations, including chest x-ray, stress test, electrocardiogram (EKG), blood pressure, vision and hearing tests, and testing for high-risk cancers. Fire and emergency service departments noted that various cancers and heart problems were identified early because of the medical exams.

Ten departments had an exercise facility at each station. Facilities featured treadmills and universal weight machines in most cases, and cross-training machines in 50 percent of the responding departments.

Less than one-third of the departments tested body fat percentages and established a body fat reduction plan. An additional five departments contracted with licensed industrial hygienists to address specific injury risks, and only two of the programs included PFTs.

Three-quarters of the departments funded the entire cost of a health and wellness program through a variety of sources. The fundraising method most commonly used to cover program costs was a local tax. In three other cases, funding was provided either directly from the employees or through worker's compensation.

UPDATE ON MODEL PROGRAM ELEMENTS FROM PREVIOUS REPORT

In the previous two versions of this Guide, published in 1992 and 2003, 14 of the 16 departments studied were featured as case studies in an attempt to help departments build their programs using the experience of other volunteer departments. Some of these departments were profiled through an IAFC initiative funded by a USFA cooperative agreement. Although not all of the components were exactly replicable, they provided benchmarks against which volunteer departments could compare their programs. Following is the current status of programs from six of the previously studied departments.

Brodhead Fire Department, Wisconsin

Beginning in 2006, the Brodhead Fire Department began taking steps to make sure that individuals joining the department meet health standards. Since that time, all new members are required to have a complete medical physical with labs, EKG stress test, hearing test, lung capacity test, and complete medical history review with a doctor that the fire department has chosen. The department has failed several applicants, but also alleviated potential problems as well as helped notify those individuals of health issues that they should address with their own medical professional. Although this medical requirement has affected its membership numbers slightly, the department would rather have fewer members who are healthy and capable of performing firefighting duties than more members who may not be physically fit for the job. The department is confident that all new members are healthy and capable of performing the demanding tasks of firefighting. The department's long-term goal is to incorporate mandatory annual physicals for all members, but this will depend on future funding.

Chesterfield County Fire and EMS, Virginia

The Chesterfield Fire and EMS Health and Fitness Program recognizes that its firefighters have different fitness needs to keep them in good condition, as members are of different ages, genders, and levels of physical fitness. The department, along with the assistance of health and fitness professionals, has developed a comprehensive fitness program that provides different levels of fitness training for uniformed members. Each quarter, the program increases intensity and focuses on specific types of fitness and cardiovascular exercises to promote continued improvement in both strength training and cardiovascular endurance.

Once a year, the members are evaluated with a fitness performance test to determine individual improvement and to focus on areas that need additional attention. These tests include flexibility, strength, cardiovascular endurance, and body fat measurements. This program is designed to improve each member's physical conditioning and wellness to help the department better perform its duties.

Hartford Emergency Services, Vermont

Hartford Emergency Services is a combination department that serves a population of 10,000. Their volunteers are paid on a per-call basis. To increase members' support, the department developed the fitness program by working with both volunteer and career firefighters.

Under the IAFF-IAFC program, they have initiated the following program components:

- Two certified peer fitness trainers work with the membership to develop individual routines and to keep logs and records.
- Fitness evaluations are conducted twice a year on all members that are in the program and exercising.
- All members of the department are given a yearly physical to determine if they are fit for duty. This physical conforms to OSHA and NFPA requirements (Health and Life Style Questionnaire, Hearing Test, Vision Test, Blood Analysis, Chest X-Ray, 12 Lead, Spirometry, Physical Exam by Doctor, and TB test).
- Health classes, lectures, and relevant literature also are offered, free of charge.
- All career personnel are required to work out for a minimum of 45 minutes every day that they are on duty. It is voluntary, yet highly encouraged, for all volunteer personnel to take part in the program as well.

Howland Fire Department, Ohio

The Howland Fire Department in Warren, Ohio, also had experienced moderate success with its health and fitness program, which it implemented in 1989. Department officials report that 95 percent of all members—up from 75 percent in the 2003 study—participate in the program in some way. Forty percent of the membership—an increase from 25 percent in the previous study—participates 3 days per week. Department officials attribute any lack of interest among members to time constraints due to increased call volume. Due to recent union contract negotiations, the contract now requires all paid members to participate in a physical fitness program.

The program includes pre-acceptance medical screening, monthly physical fitness evaluation, and cardiovascular-focused fitness equipment. To enhance the program, the department added a "jump-stretch" program, which focused on low impact stretching warm-ups to make members more flexible, and recently added an elliptical machine to their gym. Additionally, the department has paid specific attention to maintaining the fitness equipment.

Lacey Fire Department, Washington

The Lacey Fire District in Lacey, Washington, has increased the breadth and scope of its health and fitness program since its inception in the mid-1980s. In 2007, the District implemented a peer fitness program initially providing training for three members to serve as PFTs. Additionally, they provided an assortment of fitness and strength equipment for members' use in dedicated fitness space at each fire station. The fitness area and equipment is available to all members, and onduty emergency response personnel have a voluntary onduty workout time opportunity. A Division Chief is responsible for the Health and Safety program.

Most of the department's 180 members participate in the program. The program's popularity and high participation rates are attributed to the demonstrated support of the program by management and the personal commitment to fitness by the members.

Plantation Fire Department, Florida

The Plantation Fire Department in Plantation, Florida, created its health and fitness program in the early 1990s. The program incorporated a screening and evaluation component, which included full blood laboratory screenings, annual flu shots, and rehabilitation following injuries. The program also included an educational piece, with nutrition and weight management, exercise, back care, stress management, and heart disease counseling provided to members. The department purchased universal machines and stationary bicycles for all stations, and medical examinations were paid by the department.

As of 2008, Plantation Fire Department has pared down its health and fitness program, retaining only the benefits that the city provides to its employees, such as the use of exercise equipment, by membership, at three city-managed exercise facilities, and other medical and testing programs.

Plantation Fire Department officials indicated that the program's demise was mainly due to its high cost and little interest among membership. In addition, the city already provided certain benefits to all city employees and volunteers at no cost or for reasonable fees.

In: Firefighter Fitness: A Health and Wellness Guide   ISBN: 978-1-60741-650-0
Editor: Ernest L. Schneider   © 2010 Nova Science Publishers, Inc.

Chapter 5

DEVELOPMENT OF A HEALTH AND WELLNESS PROGRAM FOR VOLUNTEER FIRE AND EMERGENCY SERVICES DEPARTMENTS

U.S. Fire Administration

The previous chapters examined why health and wellness programs are essential and what departments across the Nation are doing with their programs. This chapter focuses on how a volunteer or combination department can develop a health and wellness program of its own.

The development of a health and wellness program involves both the implementation of program components and the establishment of a program administration and supporting groundwork. This chapter begins with a look at the major program components, followed by a discussion of the administration of a health and wellness program. Chapter VI brings all of the recommendations together with a step-by-step program implementation guide.

PROGRAM COMPONENTS

A comprehensive health and wellness program includes the following components:

- regular fitness screenings and medical evaluations;
- fitness program (cardiovascular, strength, and flexibility training);

- behavioral modification (smoking, hypertension, diet, cholesterol, diabetes);
- volunteer education; and
- screening volunteer applicants.

When a program combines all of these components, volunteers pay more attention to their personal health and wellness, which will improve the department overall. If a department cannot implement the entire program at once, it is far better to initiate some of these components than to do nothing.

Regular Fitness Screenings and Medical Evaluations

Regular screenings and medical evaluations are an important foundation for a successful, comprehensive health and wellness program. NFPA 1582, *Standard on Comprehensive Occupational Medical Program for Fire Departments* provides a set of guidelines for medical testing and screening, which simplifies the development of this component.

Fitness Screening. Prior to participation in any fitness program, adults should be effectively screened in accordance with American College of Sports Medicine (ACSM) Guidelines. These guidelines will classify individuals as a low, moderate, or high risk for participation in any fitness program. Individuals classified as high risk should be referred to a high-risk intervention program, closely supervised by medical personnel. These individuals will incur the greatest risk for cardiac complication and increased health care costs. They may be at risk from the exercise program itself, if it is not properly modified to their capabilities. Individuals classified as moderate risk should participate only in moderately strenuous programs without having had a medical exam within the past year. Nor should they undergo testing without medical supervision. Individuals classified as low risk can participate in an exercise program that can be vigorous in nature or undergo testing without medical supervision.

Annual Medical Examinations. The risks that confront a first responder necessitate a regular evaluation of health and wellness. Identifying risks might preclude a volunteer from riding for a period of time. In this circumstance, however, the first responder should not take this action as a punishment, but rather be aware that it is for his or her health and safety as well as that of other department members and the community they serve.

The examinations should be standardized for all members. Some departmental programs have developed partnerships with a local health practitioner who offered a discounted rate and provided standardized examinations for volunteers. Such a physician would work with the health and wellness coordinators, in addition to the members, providing a much-needed perspective on the condition of the membership in that specific department.

NFPA 1582 suggests the following items be reviewed as part of the medical examination; any problems identified should be rectified before the firefighter is allowed to respond to emergencies:[1]

- vital signs—namely pulse, respiration, blood pressure, and, if indicated, temperature;
- dermatological system;
- ears, eyes, nose, mouth, throat;
- cardiovascular system;
- respiratory system;
- gastrointestinal system;
- genitourinary system;
- endocrine and metabolic systems;
- musculoskeletal system;
- neurological system;
- audiometry;
- visual acuity and peripheral vision testing;
- pulmonary function testing;
- laboratory testing, if indicated;
- diagnostic imaging, if indicated; and
- electrocardiography, if indicated.

Although having a common practitioner would be ideal for conducting all of these tests consistently, some fire and emergency service personnel will want to use their own physician. These first responders should be provided with a common medical examination form, developed by the department, to standardize the process and to ensure comparable results.

Fitness Program

A well-designed fitness program should include both physical activity and exercise. It is designed to improve individual physical condition and endurance and to reduce the risk of heart attacks and other major problems facing firefighters and EMS personnel.

Physical activity is defined as bodily movement produced by the contraction of skeletal muscle, which increases energy expenditure—in simple language, moving around.

Exercise is planned or structured movement, repetitive in nature. It is intended to improve or maintain one or more of the following components of physical fitness:

- cardiorespiratory fitness;
- muscular strength;
- muscular endurance;
- flexibility; and
- body composition.

Exercise and training programs now have evolved beyond the simple focus of the health-related aspects of physical fitness to include the skill-related aspects vital to first responder performance. The fire service has shifted its emphasis to training programs that improve the overall quality of life by maximizing the carryover gains from training into the activities of emergency response.

Surveys indicate that about 25 percent of the American population engages in no physical activity, and an additional 37 percent undertake insufficient physical activity. Nationally, dropout rates for those beginning an exercise program are alarming, reaching 50 percent or more by the end of the first 6 months. The reasons are complex and multifaceted, influenced by factors associated with each individual, the environment, and the stage of behavioral readiness and features of the program itself.[2]

Moderate-Intensity Program. Historically, attention has focused solely on exercise, promoting its benefits and virtues. Recent research, however, has demonstrated numerous health benefits associated with regular participation in intermittent, moderate-intensity physical activity in addition to exercise. Consequently, the CDC have amended and expanded their emphasis to include greater awareness of participation in physical activity and the quantities and intensities necessary to achieve health benefits, which are lower than previously thought to be necessary. This does not discount the added benefits of more intense, longer duration exercise. There are benefits from increased activity that more people (and firefighters) may be willing to maintain.

According to former U.S Surgeon General Richard Carmona: "Significant health benefits can be obtained by including a moderate amount of physical activity on most, if not all days of the week. Through a modest increase in daily activity, most Americans can improve their health and quality of life… Additional health benefits can be gained through greater amounts of physical activity. People who maintain a regular regimen of activity that is of longer duration or of more vigorous intensity are likely to derive greater benefit."

Moderate intensity activities are equivalent to walking 3 to 4 mph (15 to 20 minutes to walk a mile). These casual daily activities are the easiest to promote and implement and are key to any successful fitness program.

Figure 2 shows how anyone can increase physical activity in his or her daily lives even while not committing to a regular workout routine.

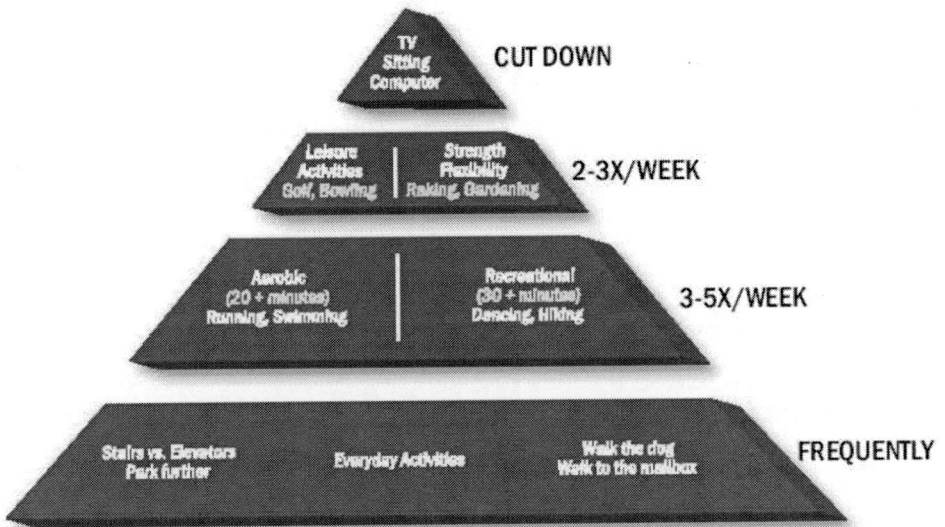

Source: Institute for Research and Education, 1996.

Figure 2. Physical Activity Pyramid.[3]

Some additional examples of moderate activity:

- washing/waxing a car (45 to 60 min);
- washing windows/floors (45 to 60 min);
- playing volleyball/touch football (45 min);
- gardening or raking leaves (30 to 45 min);
- basketball game (15 to 20 min);
- bike riding (30 min);
- moderate- to high-tempo dancing (30 min);
- swimming laps (15 to 20 min); and
- brisk walking (30 min).

Cardiovascular Program. The goals of the cardiovascular portion of the fitness program are to improve performance, improve health, prevent injury, decrease the risk of heart attack, and increase heat tolerance. The first step is to increase daily activity. Not only will this improve health, but it also creates a more positive, active image for first responders in the community.

At the next level, participants could engage in moderate intensity exercise for 30 or more minutes a minimum of three times per week. This can include such activities as a brisk walk or a bicycle ride. Firefighters and EMS personnel should set a pace with which they are comfortable and increase the pace as they wish.

As participants become comfortable with the moderate level, they could transition to a higher intensity exercise. Once again, participants set their own pace. Depending on the needs of the individual, this exercise could be performed in a gym, at the department, or at home.

It may be possible to develop partnerships with a nearby fitness center. Then, fire and emergency service personnel would have access to a wide range of equipment and fitness expertise. This can also benefit the department, as using the fitness center will reduce the time commitment for the volunteer coordinator and reduce liability concerns. On the negative side, the use of a fitness center may cost more money, be inconvenient for the volunteers, and involve more self-motivation. A more detailed discussion about developing partnerships is provided later in this chapter under Program Administration.

Exercising in a department facility can foster a sense of camaraderie among the volunteers. Team competitions and participation in community events also can provide motivation for greater participation in fitness programs. Cardiovascular exercise can be performed in the department with the aid of only a few machines. Treadmills, stationary bicycles, elliptical machines, stair climbers, and rowing machines can serve volunteer departments adequately. These machines require a modest initial cost but, in the long term they may reduce costs of membership fees to fitness centers.[4]

Strength Training. The goals of strength training are to protect against injury, improve performance, maintain the appropriate body composition, and improve health. An appropriate strength-training regimen includes a progressive weight lifting and calisthenics program. These exercises should be performed two to four times per week, working the major muscle groups twice a week.

A weight-training regimen includes a minimum of one to three sets of six to 12 repetitions each day at a comfortable weight. Individuals should begin with one set at a lower weight level and work up to three sets at a higher weight level. Participants, however, need to progress at their own pace. Ideally, the selection of exercises should emulate first responder activities for the weight training to improve job performance.

A calisthenics routine may include situps, pullups, and crunches plus a selection of exercises aimed at strengthening and stabilizing the core muscle group. Here too, participants progress at their own pace.

Weight lifting and calisthenics can be done at a fitness center, in the department, or at home. Although a fitness center offers a wide range of strength training machines, most departments could provide barbells, dumbbells, Smith presses, and weight stations at minimal costs.[5]

Flexibility Training. The goal of flexibility training is to prevent injuries, especially to the lower back. Participants engage in moderate stretching, holding each stretch for 10 to 30 seconds. Although stretching is encouraged prior to exercise or physical activity, the greatest gains in flexibility are made after exercise, when muscles are warm. Therefore, stretching should be done both as a warmup and after exercise. Strength and flexibility go hand-in-hand. Increasing both simultaneously will improve first responder performance and decrease the risk for injury.

Behavioral Modification Program

Behavioral modification is another core component of a comprehensive health and wellness program. Firefighters and emergency services personnel will want to address any preexisting health conditions and personal behaviors that heighten their risks of CVD or other injuries. CVD is by far the leading cause of firefighter deaths in the United States. Smoking, hypertension, an unhealthy diet, unmanaged cholesterol, unmanaged diabetes, and high blood glucose levels are all contributors to CVD, and each can be modified. (See Appendix B for a detailed discussion of the medical physiology of each of these contributing factors to CVD.)

Smoking. Smoking cessation is one of the most important interventions for preventing CVD. Smoking cessation reduces the risk of the first heart attack by 65 percent.[6] The strategies to reduce the risk of CVD associated with smoking are straightforward:

- Individuals can attend a smoking cessation program, employ nicotine replacement therapy, or discuss medication options with their physician. Over-the-counter and prescription medications are available to help overcome the smoking addiction.
- Departments can aggressively promote smoking cessation programs available through local hospitals and other health agencies and consider sponsoring programs for their employees.
- Departments can ban smoking among personnel at the station.
- Departments can implement regulations that protect personnel from second-hand smoke at the station.

Hypertension. Strategies to reduce the risk of CVD associated with hypertension are varied and often overlapping. The degree of risk and the appropriate interventions depend on the degree of hypertension and the presence of additional risk factors. Individuals with elevated blood pressure, even high-normal blood pressure, should consult with their physician. During the consultation, the physician needs to be made aware of the types of job stresses encountered in emergency response. The physician may recommend drug therapy to treat hypertension, but lifestyle modifications also should be used in conjunction with medication. In fact, lifestyle modifications may be sufficient to avoid medication or to prevent the need for medication.

Diet. An appropriate diet is an important factor in the prevention of CVD. In general, the three primary objectives of diet modification are

Attaining ideal body weight.
Ensuring a well-balanced diet high in fruits and vegetables.
Restricting saturated fats and simple, refined carbohydrates (sugars). In general, less than 30 percent of daily calorie intake should be from fats

(with less than 10 percent of calories coming from saturated fats). Cholesterol intake should be less than 300 mg/day. Because of growing evidence that Omega-3 fatty acids protect against CVD, it is commonly recommended that individuals eat fish one or two times per week.[7]

Lowering caloric intake is important in weight reduction. A loss of excess body fat is associated with decreased blood pressure. A 2-pound reduction in body weight is associated with a 1.6-mmHg reduction in systolic blood pressure and a 1.3-mmHg reduction in diastolic blood pressure. The higher an individual's blood pressure is, the higher the risk for CVD.[8]

Reducing salt intake is beneficial for individuals with elevated blood pressure. Sodium restriction is associated with a decrease in blood pressure in most people.[9] Salt restriction can be achieved by avoidance of salty foods (e.g., potato chips, olives), by not using or restricting the amount of salt while cooking or seasoning foods, and by avoiding processed food. Other recommended dietary changes include decreasing alcohol and caffeine consumption and increasing fruits, vegetables, and fish in the diet.

Reducing Cholesterol. As discussed in detail in Appendix B, the risk of CVD is heightened with unmanaged cholesterol. In general, the strategies for managing cholesterol levels fall into two categories: life-style modification and drug therapy. Drug therapy may be necessary for individuals who are at high risk for cardiovascular disease (risk factors discussed in Appendix B). If cholesterol levels are a concern, firefighters and emergency services personnel should consult with a physician to see which combination of strategies is right for their individual needs.

The primary lifestyle modifications that affect high cholesterol involve diet and exercise, in addition to drug therapy. In all cases, drug therapy should occur in conjunction with dietary therapy and increased physical activity. In many instances, drug treatment for high cholesterol levels is a long-term treatment strategy, and it is imperative that individuals continue to take their medication. Very often individuals will not "feel better" when they are taking the medication, but the cardiovascular system is "working better."

Managing Diabetes and Reducing Blood Glucose Levels. Diabetes often coexists with other risk factors for cardiovascular disease. Clustered, these risk factors are termed "metabolic syndrome X" and include abdominal obesity, hypertension, dyslipidemia, and an inability to use glucose effectively (diabetes). Therefore, a person with diabetes must very aggressively control other risk factors. A diabetic should lose excess body weight, exercise regularly, and eat a diet low in simple sugars and carbohydrates. Because of the complexity of the disease, its relationship to heart disease, and the difficulty controlling blood glucose levels, a diabetic person should consult regularly with a physician about a diet and exercise program and the need for medication.

Educating Membership

Education is another core component of a comprehensive health and wellness program and is an important step to shift the culture of the fire and emergency services. Education includes health (nutrition and fitness), orthopedic, and ergonomic seminars or workshops. By using interest surveys and determining needs, seminars can be tailored to include back care, nutrition, supplements, stress management, resiliency training, diet, heart disease, smoking, and injury prevention. Short seminars can be included in the department's regular training or business meetings.

Some groups or individuals within the community may be willing to conduct the seminars at little or no cost. The department might find speakers willing to volunteer their time by contacting the local YMCA, health clubs, college, Chamber of Commerce, or medical community (including hospitals).

Screening Volunteer Applicants

Another component in the health and wellness program is recruiting people with good fitness habits. Recruiting healthy individuals to serve as first responders may reduce firefighter fatalities from heart attacks and other medical conditions. Physically fit individuals also may be at less of a risk of incurring traumatic injuries. Two examples of screening processes are a wildland firefighter pack test (featured in Chapter IV) and a candidate physical agility test. Both screening processes look at the challenges that face potential first responders.

The members of the IAFF-IAFC Wellness/Fitness Task Force developed the Candidate Physical Agility Test (CPAT) to establish a nondiscriminating, fitness-based test for hiring firefighters. The CPAT is administered along with other recruiting and mentoring practices. The CPAT is comprised of eight events in which the candidate must wear a 50-pound weighted belt. (A belt is used as opposed to structural turnout gear and SCBA so as not to give an advantage to experienced firefighters seeking employment.) The eight events include

- stair climb (climbing stairs with a 25-pound simulated hose pack);
- ladder raise and extension (placing and raising ground ladder to the desired floor or window);
- hose drag (stretching and advancing hoselines, charged and uncharged);
- equipment carry (removing and carrying equipment from fire apparatus to fireground);
- forcible entry (penetrating a locked door, breaching a wall);
- search (crawling through dark areas to search for victims);
- rescue drag (victim removal from a fire building); and
- ceiling pull (pulling a ceiling to check for and locate fire extension).

Although the CPAT was designed for recruitment to career departments, it can be applied to volunteer departments as well.

PROGRAM ADMINISTRATION

The administration of a health and wellness program is crucial to its success. If the program is not made a priority or is mismanaged, members may refuse to participate. On the other hand, proper management and leadership might create a positive culture change in the department.

Health and Wellness Coordinators

NFPA 1583 recommends: "The fire chief shall appoint a health and fitness coordinator (HFC). The HFC shall:

- Be either a member of the fire department or a qualified outside agent.
- Have access to the fire department physician or other subject matter expert for consultation.
- Be the administrator of all components of the health-related fitness program.
- Act as a direct liaison between the fire department physician or other subject matter expert and the fire department.
- Act as a direct liaison to the fire department's health and safety officer."[10]

Reprinted with permission from the NFPA 1583 (2008), *Standard on Health-Related Fitness Programs for Fire Department Members,* 5.1.1—5.2.2. Copyright © 2008, National Fire Proctection Association, Quincy, MA. This reprinted material is not the complete and official position of the NFPA on the referenced subject, which is represented only by the standard in its entirety.

In short, coordinators are to be the program's advocates within the department and to be coaches for the volunteers. With proper support from the officers, especially the chief, these coordinators could change the health and wellness culture within the department. Preferably, coordinators should be trained through an accredited peer fitness-training program. They coordinate all program marketing, manage data collection, and generate monthly reports for department management.

Coordinators should be available for year-round training, programming, and consultation. They will need to divide their time between addressing individual program prescription and training, monitoring performance, task analysis, injury prevention, and administration. Depending on the size of the department, multiple coordinators might be necessary.

Liability Exposure

Liability is a major concern of volunteer departments that have health and wellness programs, and an even greater concern for those looking to start one. Although there is no way to eliminate liability, there are ways to reduce it. When creating a program, a department should work with its insurance company and its legal counsel or the community's counsel. Insurance companies address these types of concerns every day and generally are inclined to offer assistance beforehand to help prevent a claim.

More importantly, departments need to keep in mind the risks that come with not implementing a health program. With first responder injury rates high, and many injuries preventable, it is likely that implementing a program will reduce injuries and save departments money in the long run.

Funding Alternatives

Creating a full health and wellness program, as outlined in this chapter, could prove costly to a department, especially a small-budget volunteer organization. There are many opportunities to help reduce costs, receive grants to cover expenses, or forge partnerships to eliminate costs. This section looks at some of the options and alternatives in funding a health program.

USFA's guide, *Funding Alternatives for Fire and Emergency Medical Services*,[11] presents a number of ideas for funding different types of programs, including a health and wellness program. One might argue that health and wellness of firefighters and EMS personnel should be a priority and be paid for from the fire service's budget. Since the current budget may be inadequate and the probability of its increase politically uncertain, other sources of funding may need to be considered. Some ideas include

- *Fees for service.* A way to raise funds for the budget that could be set aside for a health and wellness program.

- *Grants.* Funding is available from a number of sources that could be sought to help offset the cost of the program. An opportunity that each department should look at is the USFA Assistance to Firefighters Grant (AFG) program, which is highlighted later in this section.

- *Interacting and networking.* Contact State fire and EMS offices, associations, organizations, public officials, or decisionmakers and make sure they recognize the importance of health and wellness in the fire service.

- *Foundations and corporate donations.* Large foundations, community service clubs, and corporations often provide funding or in-kind donations (such as equipment) if they believe the need is present and the program is worthwhile.

- *Partnerships.* As discussed in greater detail later in this section, partnerships can minimize costs and improve relations in the community.

- *Fundraising.* This is always a good option, and one that ensures members have invested their time into the health and wellness program. Department-sponsored events such as bingo and casino nights or raffles that are specifically targeted to raising funds for first responder health and safety are likely to be supported by the community.

No matter what method is employed, each department needs to ensure that the programs are funded and supported adequately.

Assistance to Firefighters Grant

This section is from FEMA's "Fiscal Year 2008 Assistance to Firefighters Grants Program and Application Guidance."[12] The purpose of the AFG program is to award 1-year grants directly to fire departments to enhance the safety of the public and firefighters with respect to fire and fire-related hazards. This program supports departments that lack the tools and resources necessary to protect the health and safety of the public and their firefighting personnel with respect to fire and fire-related hazards.

FEMA may award AFG funds for the purpose of establishing or expanding wellness and fitness initiatives for firefighting personnel. For the fiscal year 2008 AFG, fire department wellness/fitness activities must offer periodic health screenings, entry physical examinations, and immunizations. Applicants for grants in this activity must currently offer, or plan to use grant funds to provide, all three benefits in order to receive consideration for funding for any other initiatives under this activity. High priority also is given to formal fitness and injury prevention projects. Lower priority is given to stress management, injury/illness rehabilitation, and employee assistance.

In accordance with the recommendations of the criteria development panel, the greatest benefit will be realized by supporting applications for new wellness and fitness programs. Therefore, higher competitive ratings will be given to applicants that lack wellness/fitness programs. Applicants that already provide the three requisite benefits and wish to expand their wellness and fitness program will receive lower consideration than departments that are seeking to initiate a wellness and fitness activity. Finally, because participation is critical to achieving any benefits from a wellness/fitness activity, higher competitive ratings will be given to departments whose wellness and fitness activities mandate participation and are open to all personnel.

Eligible expenditures in the firefighter Wellness and Fitness activity include the following:

- Procurement of medical services from trained medical professionals (MDs or RNs) to ensure the firefighting personnel are physically able to carry out their duties.
- Costs for personnel, physicals, physical fitness equipment (including shipping charges and sales tax as applicable), and supplies directly related to performance of physicals or physical fitness activities. Ineligible expenditures include the following items:
  Transportation expenses.

Contractual services with anyone other than medical professionals listed above (e.g., health-care consultants, trainers, and nutritionists).

Fitness club memberships for firefighters and their families.

Cash incentives.

Noncash incentives (t-shirts or hats of nominal value, vouchers to local businesses, or time off).

Purchase of medical equipment.

Construction of facilities to house a fitness activity, such as exercise or fitness rooms, showers, etc.

Purchase of real estate.

Partnerships and Contracts. Implementing a health and wellness program can be both expensive for the fire or EMS department and time-consuming for the program coordinator. A complete program includes access to fitness machinery, health expertise, medical examinations, and inoculations. Many volunteer departments cannot easily afford this monetary commitment. Additionally, the program coordinator must have time for organizing, implementing, and tracking the various aspects of the program. To meet these challenges, departments can form mutually beneficial partnerships with outside organizations and businesses.

Some departments contract with local gyms, wellness centers, or other businesses that specialize in fitness/wellness programs. This provides firefighters and EMS personnel access to quality fitness machinery and the expertise of personal trainers and physical therapists. Many gyms offer group discounts for fire departments; this can be a relatively inexpensive method of providing the necessary space and equipment for fitness training. These arrangements can prove to be ineffective however; although fitness facilities may be available, many lack the needed support in programming for the first responders. Departments should consider forging agreements with facilities or businesses that will offer support in delivering task-specific programming that will prove most beneficial to firefighters and the department's investment. Even departments that use equipment within the department can benefit from contracting with a gym for assistance from personal trainers and physical therapists. Doing so can prevent injury and save time for the program coordinator.

Some departments have found that using gyms is inconvenient; firefighters and EMS personnel have to travel to the gym and exercise on their own time. Accessibility is a major factor that needs to be considered when forging partnerships or entering into contracts. If volunteers will not travel to the facility, there is little use in the partnership.

Departments also can form partnerships to provide medical attention to their volunteers. Some general practitioners offer discounted annual physicals by contract to the departments. In turn, the physician can advertise himself or herself as the physician for the local department. (The department could give them a certificate to that effect.) This is not only a cost-effective method of supplying annual physicals, but it enhances better coordination and consistency. Once the doctor has a list of the participating volunteers, he or she can contact them to schedule annual physicals. The doctor then is responsible for the scheduling and recordkeeping. The program coordinator need only read the doctor's summary reports to check for compliance. Contracting with a single doctor's office also provides a greater degree of uniformity in decisions of fitness for duty.

Partnerships between fire and emergency services departments and gyms or doctors can be mutually beneficial. The departments receive discounted services of a higher quality than they could provide internally. The gyms or doctors receive increased business and a positive local image. This type of relationship also can be formed on a larger scale. For instance, departments can contact groups such as the YMCA and the AHA to possibly fund and provide services to their fitness programs. Several local departments may find it beneficial to do this as a collaborative effort.

A relationship between the fire service and nonprofit organizations and the media can also offer opportunities to improve the general health of volunteer firefighters and EMS personnel. Nonprofits may be able to provide funding sources, equipment, or program guidance. Additionally, they can attract the attention of the news media, potentially shedding light on the important issue of first responder health. The current atmosphere of overwhelming support for first responders thereby can be harnessed to improve the condition of the fire and emergency services.

There are numerous other possibilities for programs between fire departments and nonprofit organizations. For instance, statistics show that heart disease is a leading cause of line-of-duty firefighter deaths. The AHA has supported departments that are trying to reduce their risk of heart disease through programming. One way to accomplish this is to challenge firefighters and EMS personnel to reach certain goals, such as a certain ideal weight or a specific amount of weekly exercise, and then ask the partner organization to provide the necessary information and materials. Challenges of this nature offer attainable goals and an opportunity for publicity.

Each department should develop a list of organizations to outreach for assistance. The type of organizations to consider contacting include

- YMCAs, health clubs, wellness centers;
- hospitals, medical offices, physical therapists;
- offices of nutritionists or dieticians;
- colleges and universities (medical centers, health departments, fitness centers);
- national health organizations (e.g., AHA);
- national service organizations (e.g., Lions, Rotary);
- fitness stores (e.g., Sports Authority, bicycle stores);
- health stores (e.g., General Nutrition Centers); and
- NVFC.

INCENTIVES FOR PARTICIPATION

Participation rates in health programs are dependent largely on the specific programs implemented and the participation incentive used. A key to increase involvement is to provide incentives for volunteer participation. Naturally, the more reasons a person has to participate, the more likely he or she is not only to join, but to engage actively in the program.

Nonincentivized programs generate poor levels of participation, but traditional "achievement awards" (e.g., workout equipment, certificates) demonstrate a 20- to 40-percent participation rate. Financial or personal incentives are most effective. Average participation, or use rates, for such incentive-based programs average 50 to 60 percent.[13] Examples of effective incentives that could be offered include

- cash or gift drawings;
- schedule priority;
- choice of firehouse duties;
- recognition at banquets or meetings; and
- financial rewards for program completion.

Departments should check local, State, and Federal guidelines regarding gaming and cash prizes/tax reporting guidelines before granting incentive prizes.

FIRED UP FOR FITNESS CHALLENGE

The Fired Up For Fitness Challenge is an interactive NVFC-created program where firefighters and EMS personnel can design and implement their individual fitness program. Participants measure personal progress by recording their physical activity and results such as weight loss, as well as compare their progress with fellow first responders across the Nation. Participants also receive rewards as they reach certain benchmarks of activity hours.

End Notes

[1] Reprinted with permission from NFPA 1582-2007, Standard on *Medical Requirements for Firefighters and Information for Fire Department Physicians*, 7.6. Copyright© 2007, National Fire Protection Association, Quincy, MA 02269. This reprinted material is not the complete and official position of the National Fire Protection Association, on the referenced subject, which is represented only by the standard in its entirety.

[2] Centers for Disease Control, 2005.

[3] Institute for Research and Education, 1996.

[4] Bentkowski, Frank. "NYC's Firefighters Strive for Fitness." *Fire Chief*, June 2003, pg. 70.

[5] Ibid.

[6] Ridker, Genest, and Libby, Op. cit.

[7] Ibid.

[8] Kaplan, N.M. "Systemic Hypertension: Mechanisms and Diagnosis." In: Braumwald, E., D.P. Zipes, and P. Libby, (eds). *Heart Disease: A Textbook of Cardiovascular Medicine*. 6th Ed. Philadelphia: W.B. Saunders, 2001.

[9] Ibid.

[10] Reprinted with permission from NFPA 1583-2008, *Health Related Fitness Programs for Firefighters*, 5.1.1—5.2.2. Copyright© 2008, National Fire Protection Association, Quincy, MA. This reprinted material is not the complete and official position of the NFPA on the referenced subject, which is represented only by the standard in its entirety.

[11] United States Fire Administration. *Funding Alternatives for Fire and Emergency Medical Services*. Oct. 2007.

[12] United States Fire Administration. *Fiscal Year 2008 Assistance to Firefighters Grants Program and Application Guidance*. Feb. 2008.

[13] Wellness Council of America. *Healthy Balance Program*. Ongoing program involving 50,000 employees from Caterpillar Inc.   Annual review, 2000.

In: Firefighter Fitness: A Health and Wellness Guide   ISBN: 978-1-60741-650-0
Editor: Ernest L. Schneider   © 2010 Nova Science Publishers, Inc.

Chapter 6

IMPLEMENTING A HEALTH AND WELLNESS PROGRAM

U.S. Fire Administration

Chapter V addressed the components and administration of a model health and wellness program for volunteer fire and emergency service departments. This chapter looks at how to combine these components into an effective program and implement the program at the department level.

The most important step in implementing a health and wellness program is planning. An effective implementation plan should address two basic areas: department planning and assessment; and data collection, analysis, and program evaluation.

DEPARTMENT PLANNING AND ASSESSMENT

As discussed in Chapter V, the foundation of an effective health and wellness program, especially for volunteers, is customizing it to meet the needs of the participants. There is no model plan that will work for all departments in all places, but there are model elements and core components that should be implemented. These elements and components were laid out in Chapter V.

Creating the Vision

When implementing a program, a small steering committee should first develop a vision for the department's program. When developing the vision for the program, the committee should identify the major issues that affect the volunteers and the impact of those issues on both the individual and department (some of the issues that affect many, if not all, volunteers were discussed in Chapters II and III). It is very important that a representative sample of the volunteers is consulted while developing the vision. The vision should provide guidance on how to develop and implement an individualized program for the department, so making sure the targeted participants have input is critical.

Implementation Steps

With a vision developed, the department could begin the program planning, implementation, and integration process. The following areas need to be addressed during this process:

Select health and wellness coordinator(s). As discussed in Chapter V, the coordinators should be the advocates and leaders within the department for the health and wellness program. The coordinators might come from the steering committee itself or be identified by the committee while developing the vision for the program.

Consult with legal counsel and insurance company. Legal counsel and insurance companies can help diminish liability of injury and risk. Additionally, some insurance companies may give the department credit for implementing a program aimed at reducing the risk of fireground injuries and deaths.

Select program components. The department should consult with a qualified medical or fitness professional in selecting the components, or pieces of each component, to ensure the program is customized for the needs of the individual department. Departments with an older volunteer base, for example, most likely will require a different program than a department with a mix of younger and older volunteers. (All of these components are discussed in much greater detail in Chapter V.)

Create a fitness component. The fitness component should address cardiovascular fitness, muscular strength and endurance, flexibility, and body composition. The fitness component could begin with a simple encouragement to increase moderate intensity activities such as walking the dog, swimming laps, or playing basketball. Over time, the department should provide opportunities for volunteer firefighters and EMS personnel to participate in more intense workouts, whether at the department or a gym.

Create a behavioral modification component. A behavioral modification component should include smoking cessation, hypertension and cholesterol reduction, and diet modification components. Behavioral modification will help to address pre-existing health conditions that heighten risks to cardiovascular health.

Include screenings and assessments before participating in a fitness program. Most experts agree that prior to participation in any fitness program, individuals should be screened and assessed to determine risk and workout needs.

Include a regimen of regular fitness health screenings and annual medical evaluations. Volunteers should receive annual medical evaluations. In several cases, departments that have instituted a physical program discovered potentially serious health issues, and the problems were corrected before they grew serious.

Table 5. Health and Wellness Program Data.[1]

Area	Objective	Measures/Data	Collection Method	Data Sources	Area
Reaction & Satisfaction	Accessibility Effectiveness Appropriate Delivery	Perception Willingness to Participate Attitude owards programs	uestionnaire/ Survey	Participants	End of session End of program
Learning	Comprehension Retention	Self-test scores Session completion	Quizzes	Participants	During session End of session
Application & Implementaion (behavioral change impact)	Completion of programs Review of program reports Postprogram participation	Goal setting and achievement Program adheance	Followup questionnaire Observation of completed assignments	Participants Coordinators	End of session End of program 6 months postprogram
Application & Implementaion (behavioral change impact)	Volunteers regularly working out Increased endurance Postprogram participation	Goal setting and achievement Program adhernce	Fitness screenings Followup Questionnaire Observations	Participants Coordinators	End of session End of program 6 months postprogram
Financial Impact	Decreased claims Decreased absences Decreased disability	Health care premiums Total Hours (medical leave)	Firefighter observation & attendance Overtime costs	Administrtrion ShiftLeaders Chiefs/Asst. Chiefs	Monthly Quarterly

Adapted from: The Human Resources Scorecard.

Educate firefighters and emergency services personnel about health risks, nutrition, fitness, and other wellness topics. Education is one of the most important steps that a department can take to help change the health and wellness culture.

Identify department facility needs. If a department chooses to have the fitness equipment in the facility, a review of the space requirements for each piece of equipment (including electrical outlets, floor support needed, etc.) needs to be completed. Even if a department chooses to partner with a gym, the coordinators might want a bulletin board to advertise program components, a shelf or closet to keep program materials, and a file cabinet to hold program files. These facility needs are important and must be considered early in the planning process.

Develop the program budget. Creating a health and wellness program most likely will prove quite costly, which makes it a challenge, especially for smaller volunteer departments. The steering committee, or coordinators, should develop a realistic budget that funds the purchase of any startup supplies and equipment; the implemented program components, any rewards and incentives, as well as additional funding for unforeseen expenditures.

Identify funding sources. Chapter V gives several options to fund a health and wellness program without draining the department's general fund. Possible sources to cover or diminish costs include grants, in-kind donations, foundation or corporation donations, partnerships, or a general fundraising drive.

Devise marketing strategies for participation. First responders must be convinced that they should invest their free time and energy into a health and wellness program when they are already volunteering time to the department. Ideas to consider when developing marketing strategies include offering incentives (discussed in Chapter V) and discussing the importance of participation (discussed in Chapters II and III).

Make health and wellness a priority. Once the components have been selected and the program is implemented, health and wellness needs to be made a priority to fully integrate the program into the culture of the volunteers. If department leadership and health and wellness coordinators are actively advocating participation (in both words and actions), the volunteers will see that the department has identified health and wellness as a priority and will be more likely to participate.

DATA COLLECTION, ANALYSIS, AND EVALUATION

Once the program is underway, health and wellness coordinators need to review the program continuously and make changes as needed. To determine what changes are needed, coordinators will need to collect data and feedback actively from membership on a regular basis. Table 5 looks at different areas that should be evaluated, how to collect the data, and what the data state about the program.

EVALUATING PROGRAM EFFECTIVENESS

This section has been adapted from the USFA's *Fire and Emergency Services Ergonomics - A Guide for Understanding and Implementing an Ergonomics Program in Your Department,* Chapter 10, "Evaluating Program Effectiveness."[2]

In many industries, management frequently assesses the success or failure of a program through economic measures:

- Increased net production (efficiency due to lower number of quality control rejects).
- Reduced incidence of days lost.
- Reduced medical insurance cost.
- Reduced worker's compensation cost.
- Increased esprit de corps.

As can be seen, all but the first of the items on the above list apply to firefighting and EMS. A successful program anywhere must show a measurable reduction in injuries, severity of injuries, and work time loss after the program is put into place.

Measuring the effectiveness of health and wellness programs in the fire service may require the development of new criteria. In the long term, the effectiveness of a health and wellness program may be measured mostly at the local level, regardless of the size of the department, by the criteria below.

Health Statistics
- reduced injury rate;
- reduced injury severity;
- reduced overhead costs;
- reduced medical/workers' compensation costs; and
- reduced time loss.

Program Statistics
- increasing participation by membership in all aspects of program;
- number of injuries or illnesses identified by screenings; and
- hours logged by membership in physical fitness.

General
- better fitness equipment developed/purchased;
- improved eating practices;
- regular health screenings and examinations; and
- regular educational events.

With the data collected and analyzed on a regular basis, department coordinators and leadership can make smart choices about the direction, funding level, and impact of the program. Every program is a work in progress, and a health and wellness program will be no different. The key to maintaining a robust health and wellness program is adapting to the needs of the volunteers who participate. Analysis of collected data and information is the key to the success of any program.

APPENDIX A: HEALTH AND WELLNESS RESOURCES

(All contacts listed alphabetically)

Program Development Contacts

American College of Sports Medicine
Phone: 317-637-9200
Email:publicinfo@acsm.org
www.acsm.org

IAFF/IAFC Fire Service Joint Labor Management Wellness-Fitness Initiative
http://www.iaff.org/hs/Well/wellness.html

IAFC Wellness Initiative
Vicki Lee, Program Manager, IAFC
Phone: 571-221-2813
Email: vlee@iafc.org

National Fire Protection Association
Phone: 617-770-3000
www.nfpa.org

National Volunteer Fire Council
Phone: 888-ASK-NVFC (275-6832)
Email: nvfcoffice@nvfc.org

FEMA Assistance to Firefighters Grant Program
Phone: 866-274-0960
Email: usfagrants@fema.gov

USFA Firefighter Fitness and Wellness Program
www.usfa.fema.gov/fire-service/health/health.shtm

Fire Department Contacts

Austin Fire Department
1621 Festival Beach Road
Austin, Texas 78702
Phone: 512-974-0200
www.ci.austin.tx.us/fire
(Career)

Bernalillo County Fire and Rescue
6840 2nd Street N.W.
Albuquerque, New Mexico 87107
Phone: 505-761-4225
www.bernco.gov/live/departments.asp?dept=2332

(Combination)
Brodhead Fire Department
1100 West 3rd Avenue
Brodhead, Wisconsin 53520
Phone: 608-897-2112
www.cityofbrodheadwi.us/Home.cfm?DepartmentID=2
(Volunteer)

Caldwell Fire and Rescue
310 South 7th Avenue
Caldwell, Idaho 83605
Phone: 208-455-3032
www.city.cityofcaldwell.com/index.v3page?p=32337
(Volunteer)

Calgary Fire Department
4124 11th Street, SE
Calgary, Alberta, Canada T2G 3H2
Phone: 403-287-4299
http://content.calgary.ca/CCA/City+Hall/Business+Units/Calgary+Fire
+Department/index.htm
(Career)

Charlotte Fire Department
600 E. 4th Street
Charlotte, North Carolina 28202
Phone: 704-432-1654
www.charmeck.org/Departments/Fire/home.htm
(Career)

Chesterfield Fire and EMS
P.O. Box 40
Chesterfield, Virginia 23832-0040
Phone: 804-748-1360
www.co.chesterfield.va.us/PublicSafety/Fire/default.asp
(Volunteer)

Fairfax County Fire and Rescue Department
4100 Chain Bridge Road

Fairfax, Virginia 22030
Phone: 703-246-3970
www.fairfaxcounty.gov/fr/
(Combination)

Gates Fire District
2355 Chili Avenue
Gates, New York 14624
Phone: 585-426-2720
http://www.gatesfd.org/
(Volunteer)

Hartford Emergency Services
812 VA Cutoff Road
White River Jct., Vermont 05001
Phone: 802-295-3232
www.hartford.gov/EmergencyServices/default.htm
(Combination)

Los Angeles County Fire Department
464 W. 8th Street
Claremont, California 91711
Phone: 323-881-2371
www.fire.lacounty.gov/
(Career)

Miami-Dade County Fire and Rescue
9300 N.W. 41st Street
Miami, Florida 33178
Phone: 786-331-4278
www.miamidade.gov/MDFR/
(Combination)

New York City Fire Academy
Randall's Island
New York, New York 10035
Phone: 718-784-6510
www.nyc.gov/html/fdny/html/units/fire_academy/fa_index.shtml
(Career)

Phoenix Fire Department
10102 North 173rd Avenue
Waddell, Arizona 85355
Phone: 602-262-6297
http://phoenix.gov/FIRE/
(Career)

Seattle Fire Department
301 2nd Avenue, South
Seattle, Washington 98104
Phone: 206-386-1450
www.seattle.gov/fire/
(Career)

NATIONAL RESOURCES

Diet

American Dietetic Association
1-800-877-0877
www.eatright.org

Center for Nutrition Policy and Promotion
703-305-7600
www.cnpp.usda.gov

Disabilities/Injuries

American Paralysis Association
1-800-225-0292
www.christopherreeve.org

American Medical Rehab Providers
1-800-368-3513
www.amrpa.org

American Speech-Language Hearing Association
1-800-638-8255
www.asha.org

Brain Injury Association
1-800-444-6443
www.biausa.org

National Easter Seal Society
1-800-221-6827
www.easterseals.com

Disease

Alcohol and Drug Hotline
1-800-821-4357
www.highlandridgehospital.com

American Cancer Society Response Line
1-800-227-2345
www.cancer.org

American Diabetes Association
1-800-232-3472
www.diabetes.org

American Liver Foundation Hepatitis Hotline
1-800-223-0179
www.liverfoundation.org

Arthritis Foundation Information Line
1-800-283-7800
www.arthritis.org

Asthma and Allergy Foundation of America
1-800-727-8462
www.aafa.org

CDC National AIDS Hotline
1-800-342-2437
www.cdc.gov/hiv

CDC National STD Hotline
1-800-227-8922
www.cdc.gov/STD

National Foundation for Depressive Illness
1-800-248-4344
www.depression.org

National Parkinson Foundation, Inc.
1-800-327-4545
www.parkinson.org

Fitness

Aerobics and Fitness Association of America
1-800-233-4886
www.afaa.com

American College of Sports Medicine
1-800-445-4808
www.acsm.org

American Heart Association
1-800-AHA-USA-1
(800-242-8721)
www.americanheart.org

Healthier US
1-800-336-4797
www.healthierus.gov

Fire and Emergency Services

International Association of Fire Chiefs
703-273-0911
www.iafc.org

International Association of Fire Fighters
202-737-8484
www.iaff.org

National Volunteer Fire Council
1-888-ASK-NVFC
(1-888-275-6832)
www.nvfc.org

United States Fire Administration
301-447-1000
www.usfa.dhs.gov

APPENDIX B: RELATIONSHIP BETWEEN CARDIOVASCULAR RISK FACTORS AND PHYSICAL FITNESS

Cardiovascular disease (CVD) is the leading cause of death in the United States, accounting for approximately 650,000 deaths per year.[3] CVD also exacts a considerable toll on the fire and emergency services. As seen in Figure B-1, approximately 40 to 45 percent of all line-of-duty deaths among firefighters, from 1991 to 2002, were due to heart attacks, whereas less than 10 percent are due to burn injuries.[4] The USFA and the NFPA record the number of deaths and disability of firefighters due to CVD, provided the cardiac event occurred while the individual was on duty.[5, 6] It is difficult to compare the incidence of CVD in the fire and emergency services with that of the general population. (There currently is epidemiological data that indicate rate of CVD deaths in the general population, but there is no information for firefighters because no agency collects data on firefighter deaths, unless they occur in the line of duty.)

A goal of the NVFC and USFA is to make a drastic reduction in the number of firefighter deaths due to heart attacks. A commitment to health and safety also will require the fire and emergency services to continue to address line-of-duty deaths due to other causes (e.g., accidents, entrapment, thermal injuries) through training, the provision of adequate resources, and other measures.

Firefighters are most effective in their emergency response activities when they possess a thorough understanding of the nature of their profession. This appendix provides information to first responders about CVD and the risk factors associated with developing CVD. The appendix describes the prevalence and progression of CVD, including occlusion, atherosclerosis, atherosclerotic plaque and plaque rupture, and clot formation.

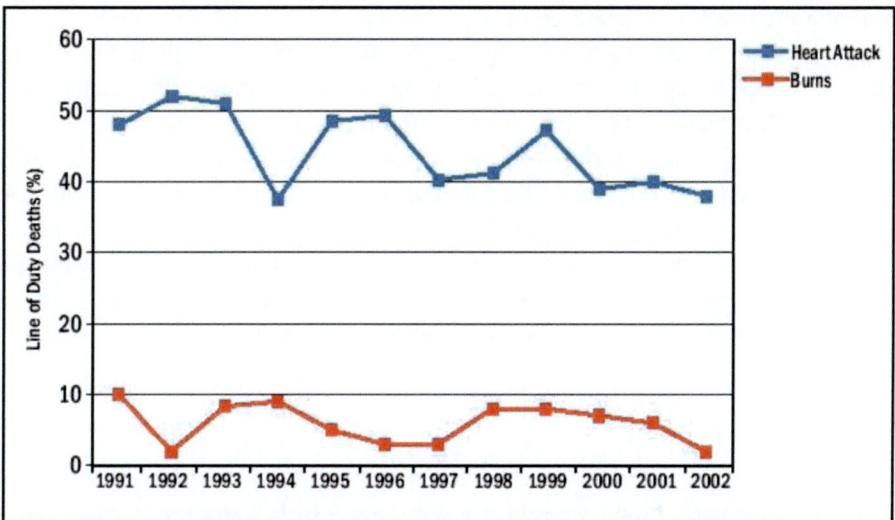

Sources: USFA, **"Firefighter Fatality Retrospective Study,"** April 2002. NFPA Firefighter Fatality Reports 2001 and 2002. NFPA Journal July/August 2002, 2003.

Figure B-1. Line-of-Duty Death by Cause.[7, 8, 9]

Finally, and perhaps most importantly, this appendix identifies the risk factors for CVD including smoking, hypertension (high blood pressure), hypercholesterolemia (high cholesterol levels), diabetes or impaired glucose tolerance, obesity, and physical activity. The more risk factors that an individual has, the greater the likelihood that he or she will suffer from CVD.

The Progression of Cardiovascular Disease

"Cardiovascular disease" refers collectively to a state of disease in the blood vessels. If blood vessels become narrowed (i.e., by the buildup of plaque) or obstructed (i.e., by a blood clot), then blood, and the oxygen and nutrients it carries, cannot be delivered to the vital organs of the body. If blood supply to the brain is impeded, a stroke occurs. If blood flow to the heart muscle is impeded, a heart attack occurs. The terms "coronary heart disease" (CHD) and "coronary artery disease" (CAD) describe specific forms of CVD in which the blood vessels supplying the heart muscle are blocked.

When there is an obstruction in a coronary vessel, the tissue below the blockage does not get adequate oxygen. If the lack of oxygen (called ischemia) is too severe, the heart tissue dies (called an infarction; a myocardial infarction means death of heart muscle tissue). Thus, a person who has suffered a myocardial infarction (also called a heart attack) has had a portion of the heart tissue destroyed. If the area supplied by the blood vessel is very small, the person may recover from the heart attack or may not even know that he or she has suffered a heart attack. However, if the area below the occlusion is too great, the heart cannot continue to function as an effective pump and death results.

Causes of Occlusion

When a coronary blood vessel (or any blood vessel) becomes blocked, tissue will be deprived of oxygen and die. The two primary causes of blockage are atherosclerosis (buildup of plaque) and a thrombus (blood clot). In reality, it appears that these causes interact; the buildup of plaque in an artery makes it more likely that a blood clot will develop. The initial buildup of plaque, which may begin in the late teens or early twenties, causes the arterial wall to become enlarged. Plaque buildup progressively decreases the size of the arterial opening until little or no blood can pass through the artery. Furthermore, the rupture of a plaque is likely to initiate the formation of a blood clot.

Atherosclerosis. Atherosclerosis refers to the disease condition in which plaque builds up in the arterial wall, which narrows the vessel opening. To fully understand how atherosclerosis develops, it is first necessary to understand the structure of an artery. Far from being a simple vessel through which blood flows, an artery is a complicated structure that plays an important role in blood clotting (or preventing blood clotting) and that constantly changes size to meet the demands of the tissue it supplies.

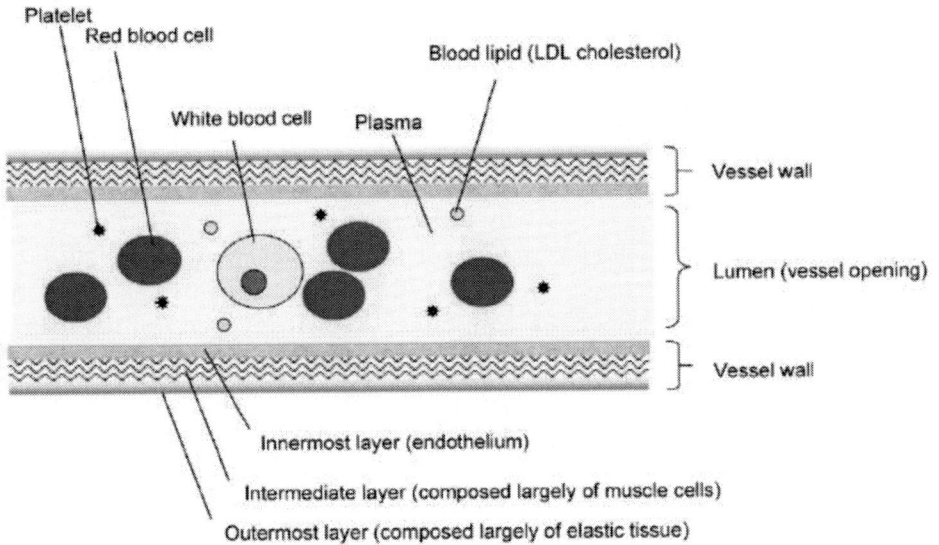

Figure B-2. Structure of a Normal Artery and Components in the Blood.

Figure B-2 is a schematic of a healthy artery. The vessel has three distinct layers. The innermost layer is composed primarily of a single layer of cells called the endothelium, and under normal conditions the endothelium plays a critical role in preventing blood clots.

The intermediate layer (tunica media) contains smooth muscle that permits the artery to change diameter to meet the needs of a tissue. For instance, when a firefighter is involved in strenuous fire suppression activities, smooth muscles around the arteries in muscles relax so that the vessel becomes larger and allows more blood to be supplied to the muscles. The outermost layer (adventia) contains connective tissue and nerves. Within the artery is the plasma (fluid portion of blood) that contains nutrients, oxygen, and blood lipids (including low-density lipoproteins). The blood vessel also contains red blood cells (RBCs), white blood cells (WBCs), and platelets.

Development of Atherosclerotic Plaque. The initiation of atherosclerotic plaque buildup may begin quite early in life; there is strong evidence that it begins in the early twenties for many people in Western, developed countries. Therefore, it is important to think of CVD as a long-term disease that begins early in life, although symptoms often are delayed until middle or older age. Also, it must be stressed that CVD may become very advanced without symptoms. In many individuals, the first sign of CVD is a fatal heart attack, thus reinforcing the need for young first responders to take steps to avoid or delay atherosclerosis. It also suggests that those in their forties and fifties should begin to address the health issues of CVD seriously even if they are symptom free.

The plaque contains a lipid-rich core, composed largely of fat, and is covered by a fibrous cap. The events in the development of atherosclerotic plaque are very complex and are described only briefly below.

The first step in the initiation of atherosclerosis is damage to the endothelium, the smooth layer of cells that line the blood vessel and is in contact with the blood. Damage may occur due to high blood pressure, chemicals from inhaled cigarette smoke, or infection. Damage to the endothelium causes or allows cholesterol, specifically low-density lipoproteins (LDLs) to move into the wall of·· the blood vessel. The presence of LDLs in the arterial wall leads WBCs, especially macrophages, to move into the arterial wall. The macrophages ingest the LDLs and become known as foam cells. Foam cells release chemicals that stimulate smooth muscle to grow and divide in the arterial wall. The additional smooth muscle in the arterial wall causes other material to accumulate in the vessel wall, thus causing the atherosclerotic plaque to grow. In later stages, the plaque may become calcified. The end result is a fatty lesion that contains a core that is rich in lipids (LDL) and dead or dying cells and a fibrous cap.

Plaque Rupture and Clot Formation. The body has a highly complicated mechanism that balances the need to keep blood in the liquid state under normal conditions with the need to produce blood clots quickly when faced with a damaged blood vessel. It appears that most cases of acute heart attack are "triggered" when an atherosclerotic plaque is disrupted, causing the development of a clot (thrombus). As depicted in Figure B-3, the clot occurs because the disruption of the plaque exposes platelet and blood coagulatory factors to underlying tissue, such as the smooth muscle and connective tissue in the vessel walls that do not possess the anticlotting factors that intact endothelium does. Exposure of the blood to underlying tissue causes the platelets to adhere to one another and form a platelet plug. The platelet plug is then reinforced by strands of thrombin to form a clot. A clot may be small enough that it does not occlude an artery, in which case the person may or may not exhibit symptoms. Conversely, the clot may be large enough to block an artery, causing a heart attack. When a plaque ruptures, it may also release a "fatty embolism," meaning a traveling fat clot that occludes an artery.

Risk Factors for Developing Cardiovascular Disease

Although it is useful to understand how CVD develops, it is more important to understand what predisposes an individual to develop CVD, and what measures can be taken to reduce the risk of developing CVD. A risk factor is a characteristic that is present early in life and is associated with an increased risk of developing future disease. A modifiable risk factor is a risk factor that can be minimized by diet, exercise, or personal habits. Table B-1 presents several risk factors for CVD, both nonmodifiable and modifiable risks. Men are more likely to suffer CVD at a younger age than females; thus, being over 45 years is considered a risk factor for males and being over 55 years is a risk factor for females. Family history is defined as the premature death (before 55 years for males or before 65 years for females) of a parent or sibling from CVD.

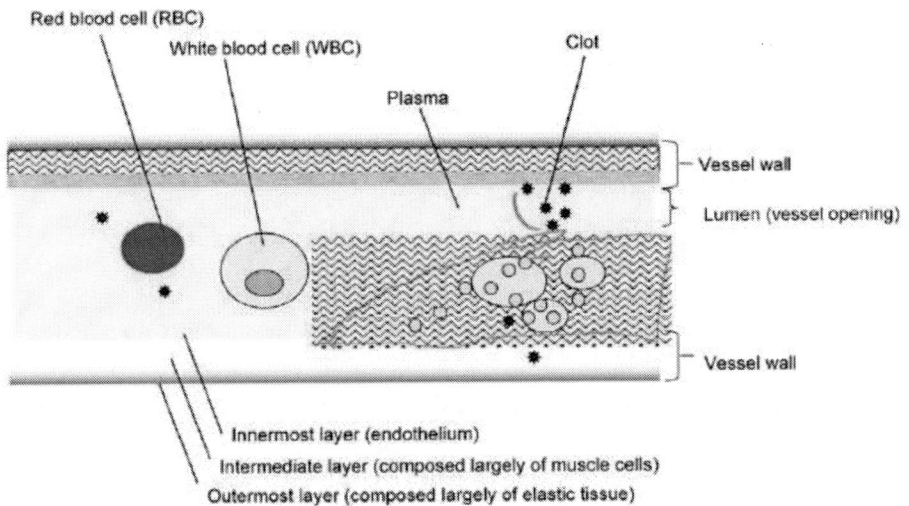

Figure B-3. Rupture of Atherosclerotic Plaque and Clot Formation.

Table B-1. Risk Factors for Developing Cardiovascular Disease

Risk Factors That Cannot be Modified	Risk Factors That Can be Modified
• Age • Heredity • Race • Gender	• Cholesterol-lipid fractions • Cigarette smoking • Diabetes mellitus • Hypertension • Obesity • Physical inactivity

Modifiable risk factors deserve a great deal of attention because it is through altering these risk factors that a person can influence his or her likelihood of developing CVD. There are six major modifiable risk factors: smoking, hypertension (high blood pressure), hypercholesterolemia (high cholesterol levels), diabetes or impaired glucose tolerance, obesity, and physical activity. The more risk factors an individual has, the greater the likelihood that he or she will suffer from CVD. The good news is that armed with information and supported by coworkers and family, most firefighters can reduce their risk for CVD by following reasonable guidelines for healthy living.

Risk Associated with Smoking

Approximately 21 percent of the adult population in the United States smokes, and approximately 4,000 young people begin to smoke each day.[10] Cigarette smoking accounts for an estimated 438,000 deaths per year in the United States, more than 20 percent of them due to CVD.[11] In fact, as early as 1983, the Surgeon General had established smoking as the leading avoidable cause of CVD. Thus, the cessation of cigarette smoking is one of the single most important interventions that can be undertaken to decrease the risk of premature death due to CVD. Smoking increases the risk for sudden cardiac death, aortic aneurysm, peripheral vascular disease, and stroke. Smoking one pack of cigarettes per day doubles the risk of CVD compared to not smoking, and smoking more than one pack triples the risk.[12, 13] Chemicals in cigarettes stimulate the sympathetic nervous system, causing an increase in heart rate and blood pressure. Carbon monoxide binds to hemoglobin, thus reducing hemoglobin's ability to carry oxygen.

As seen in Figure B-4, as the number of cigarettes smoked increases, so does the risk of coronary artery disease and stroke. "CAD Mortality," as depicted on the Y-axis in the figure, represents coronary artery disease (or coronary heart disease) mortality. A CAD mortality of 1.0 implies the same death rate as a nonsmoker.

Smoking accelerates the process of plaque development by damaging the endothelium, enhancing lipid accumulation in the arterial wall, increasing inflammation in the arterial wall, and enhancing the movement of white blood cells (especially macrophages) into the arterial wall. Simultaneously, smoking increases the likelihood of developing a blood clot by increasing platelet activation and making them more likely to adhere to each other and form a clot.

Benefits of Smoking Cessation. The good news is that much of the damage done by smoking is reversible. Smoking cessation is the single most important intervention for preventing cardiovascular death. Encouragingly, smoking cessation reduces the risk of the first heart attack by 65 percent.[15]

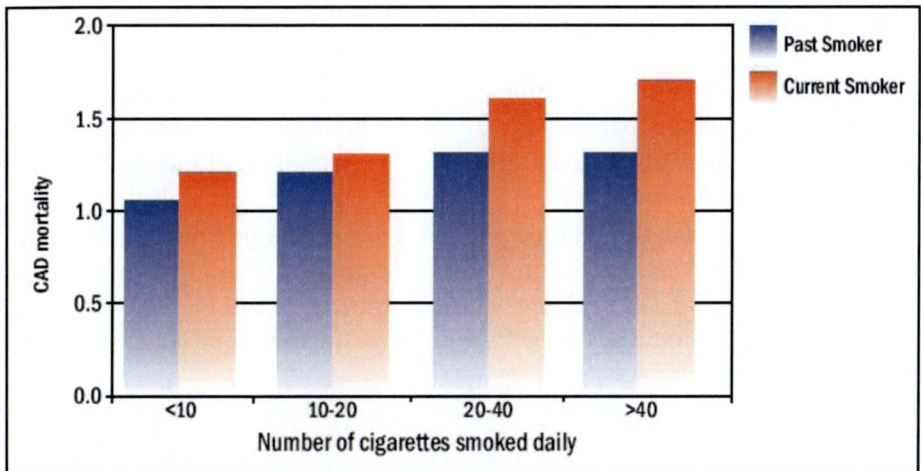

Source: "The Health Benefits of Smoking Cessation: A Report from the Surgeon General," 1990.

Figure B-4. Coronary Artery Disease and Stroke Versus Cigarette Smoking in Current and Past Smokers.[14]

Strategies for Smoking Cessation. The strategies to reduce the risk of CVD associated with smoking are straightforward:

- Quit smoking, and encourage fellow first responders to quit smoking. Individuals wanting to quit smoking should consider attending a smoking cessation program, nicotine replacement therapy (nicotine chewing gum), or discuss medication options with their physician. There are over-the-counter and prescription medications available to help overcome the smoking addiction.
- Fire and emergency service departments should aggressively promote smoking cessation programs available through local hospitals and other health agencies and consider sponsoring programs for their employees.
- Departments should consider policies that ban smoking among first responders.
- Departments should have regulations that protect first reponders from secondhand smoke.

Risk Associated with Hypertension

Hypertension refers to a chronic, persistent elevation of blood pressure. Hypertension is actually defined as the level of blood pressure that is associated with a twofold increase in long-term risk of mortality.[16] Table B-2 presents various blood pressure categories. Epidemiological data show that the risk of death doubles with a systolic blood pressure greater than or equal to 140 mmHg and a diastolic blood pressure of greater than or equal to 90; and a blood pressure above 140/90 is defined as hypertension. However, as seen in Figure B-5, the risk of developing CVD increases directly with increasing levels of both systolic and diastolic blood pressure.

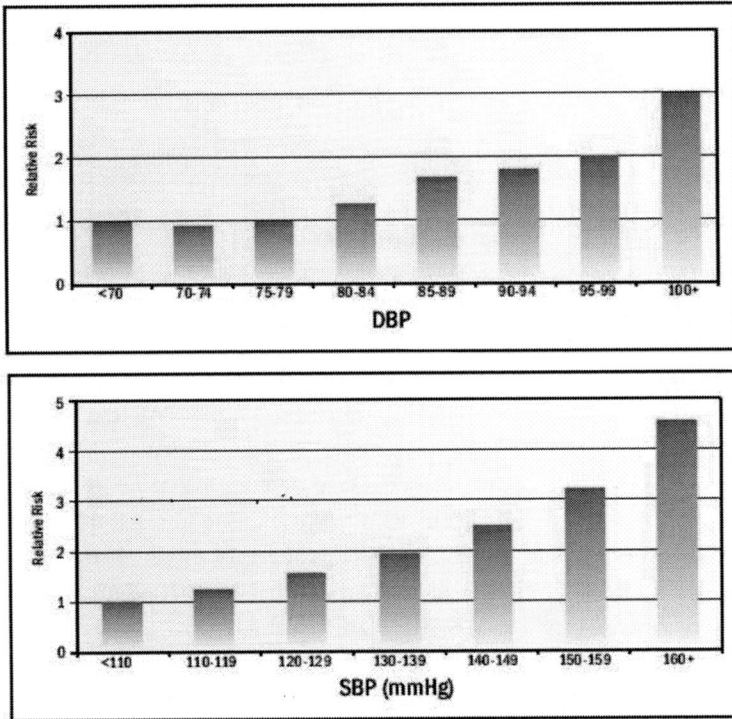

Source: National Blood Pressure Education Program Working Group. Arch. Intern Med., 1993.

Figure B-5. Relative Risk of Cardiovascular Disease Versus Blood Pressure.[17]

Table B-2. Classification of Blood Pressure—Adults (Not on Blood Pressure Medications)

Category	Blood Pressure (mmHg)		
	Systolic		Diastolic
Optimal	<120	and	<80
Normal	<130	and	<85
High-Normal	130-139	and	<85

Table B-2. (Continued)

Category	Blood Pressure (mmHg)		
	Systolic		**Diastolic**
Hypertension			
Stage 1	140-159	or	90- 99
Stage 2	160-179	or	100-109
Stage 3	≥180	or	≥100

Role of Hypertension in Cardiovascular Disease. Hypertension accelerates the atherosclerotic progress by damaging the lining of the blood vessels (endothelium). If untreated, approximately 50 percent of patients with hypertension die from coronary heart disease or congestive heart failure, another 33 percent die from stroke, and 10 to 15 percent die due to renal failure.

Reducing blood pressure levels decreases the risk of CVD. In fact, a 5- to 6-mmHg reduction in diastolic blood pressure or a 10-mmHg reduction in systolic blood pressure decreases the risk of cardiovascular disease by as much as 40 percent.[18]

Hypertension could be slowed, and possibly prevented, by preventing obesity, moderate reduction in salt intake, higher levels of physical activity, and avoidance of excessive alcohol consumption.[19]

Strategies for Controlling Hypertension. The strategies to reduce the risk of CVD associated with hypertension are varied and often overlapping. Furthermore, the degree of risk and the appropriate interventions depend upon the degree of hypertension and the presence of additional risk factors. If you have elevated blood pressure, or even high-normal blood pressure, you should consult with your physician. Make sure he or she knows the types of job stresses you encounter as you discuss controlling your blood pressure. Table B-3 presents recommendations for treatment based on the level of blood pressure and the presence of additional risk factors. This table should serve as a basis for discussions with your physician regarding how to best control your blood pressure given your overall medical condition. Although your physician may recommend drug therapy to treat hypertension, lifestyle modifications should be used in conjunction with medication. Furthermore, lifestyle modifications may be sufficient to avoid medication or to prevent the need for medication. If, however, your physician has prescribed a medication, you should take it faithfully.

Lifestyle Modifications. The primary lifestyle modifications to help reduce hypertension include smoking cessation, diet, and exercise, with the overall goals of losing weight, increasing physical activity levels, and decreasing salt intake. Lifestyle modifications also may be appropriate for those who are currently in the normal range because blood pressure tends to increase with age. Therefore, it is prudent to take steps to control blood pressure before it becomes a problem. The benefits of lifestyle modifications are readily apparent when one realizes that even modest reductions in blood pressure translate into significant reductions in the risk of cardiovascular disease.

Table B-3. General Guidelines for Strategies to Reduce or Treat Blood Pressure Based on Blood Pressure Readings and Presence of Additional Risk Factors

Blood Pressure Category	No Other Risk Category	At Least One Other Risk Factor (Not Including Diabetes)	Diabetes and Clinical Evidence of Heart Disease
High-normal	Lifestyle modification	Lifestyle modification	Drug therapy
Stage 1	Lifestyle modification	Lifestyle modification	Drug therapy
Stages 2 and 3	Drug therapy	Drug therapy	Drug therapy

Diet. A decrease in total caloric intake is important in weight reduction. A loss of excess body fat is associated with decreased blood pressure. A two-pound reduction in body weight is associated with a 1.6 mmHg reduction in systolic blood pressure and a 1.3 mmHg reduction in diastolic blood pressure.[20]

A reduction in salt intake is beneficial for individuals with elevated blood pressure. Sodium restriction is associated with a decrease in blood pressure in most people.[21] Salt restriction can be achieved by avoidance of salty foods (i.e., potato chips, olives, etc.), by not using additional salt while cooking or seasoning foods, and by avoiding processed food.

Other recommended dietary changes include a decrease in alcohol and caffeine consumption, and an increase in fruits, vegetables, and fish in the diet.

Types of Lipids

Blood lipids are comprised primarily of triglycerides and cholesterol. Triglycerides are composed primarily of fatty acids and are the type of fat ingested in food. Cholesterol also is ingested in food, but in much smaller amounts than triglycerides. Cholesterol is important for cell membranes and hormone synthesis, but when present in excessive amounts, it can have negative health outcomes. Cholesterol and triglycerides are carried in the blood by a lipoprotein molecule. Low-density lipoproteins (LDLs), also known as "bad cholesterol", and high-density lipoproteins (HDLs), also known as "good cholesterol", vary in their densities and in the way they transport cholesterol.

An analysis of blood lipids that includes LDLs and HDLs provides important information (in addition to total cholesterol) regarding an individual's risk for cardiovascular disease. As seen in Table B-4, elevated levels of triglycerides, cholesterol, and LDL-cholesterol are associated with increased risk of CVD. On the other hand, increased levels of HDL-cholesterol are associated with a decreased risk of cardiovascular disease. Therefore, elevated levels of HDL are desirable. In fact, high HDL levels represent a lowered risk of cardiovascular disease.

Table B-4. Description of Various Lipids and Their Relationship to Cardiovascular Disease

Type of Lipid	Description	Relationship to CVD
Triglyceride	Simple fat, found in food	Positive relationship. As LDL levels increase, so does the risk of CVD.
Cholesterol	A derived fat that is essential for cell function and hormone production but is detrimental in excessive amounts	Positive relationship. As LDL levels increase, so does the risk of CVD.
Low-density lipoprotein (LDL cholesterol)	"Bad cholesterol." These lipoproteins transport concentrated amounts of cholesterol to the arterial wall where it contributes to plaque buildup. These lipoproteins contain a large portion of cholesterol.	Positive relationship. As LDL levels increase, so does the risk of CVD.

Table B-4. (Continued)

Type of Lipid	Description	Relationship to CVD
High-density lipoprotein (HDL cholesterol)	"Good cholesterol." These lipoproteins pick up cholesterol in the bloodstream and transport it from the arteries to the liver, where it is metab-olized. These lipoproteins contain a small portion of cholesterol.	Negative relationship. As HDL levels increase, the risk of CVD decreases, making high HDLs a negative risk factor

Because high levels of some lipids (triglycerides, total cholesterol, or LDL-cholesterol) are undesirable and low levels of other lipids (HDL-cholesterol) are undesirable, the term hyperlipidemia (high lipid levels) is not always appropriate. Instead, medical professionals prefer the term dyslipidemia (altered or dysfunctional levels of lipids in the blood) to describe lipid disorders that may include values that are too high (for triglycerides, total cholesterol, or LDL-cholesterol) or too low (for HDL-cholesterol).

Cholesterol

High cholesterol levels (hypercholesterolemia) increase the risk of CVD. Elevated levels of cholesterol in young adults greatly increase their risk of coronary heart disease later in life. In fact, young men who are in the upper quartile (highest 25 percent for cholesterol levels) have a ninefold increase in risk of heart attack compared to men in the lowest quartile (lowest 25 percent).[22]

As seen in Table B-5, desirable levels of cholesterol are less than 200 mg/dL, whereas high cholesterol is defined as total cholesterol above 240 mg/dL of blood. There is a twofold increase in risk of cardiovascular mortality when cholesterol levels are elevated to 240 mg/dL versus 200 mg/dL. Unfortunately, approximately half of American adults have cholesterol values greater than 200 mg/dL, and about 20 percent have values above 240 mg/dL.[23] The increase in risk of CVD increases progressively with increasing levels of cholesterol; there is a 20- to 30-percent increase in risk for coronary heart disease for every 10 mg/dL increase in cholesterol.[24] Although values above 240 mg/dL are defined as high, it is important to note that the risk of coronary heart disease increases in a curvilinear fashion with increasing levels of total cholesterol. The 10-year risk of coronary heart disease increases as the total cholesterol level increases.[25] The risk of coronary heart disease associated with increasing total cholesterol levels is affected by the presence of other risk factors.

Table B-5. Classification of Lipid Levels[26]

Lipid (classification)	Value (mg/dL)
Total cholesterol	
Desirable	<200
Borderline	200-239
High	>240
LDL-cholesterol	
Optimal	<100
Near optimal	100-129
Borderline High	130-159
High	160-189
Very High	>190
HDL-cholesterol	
Low	<40
High	>60
Triglyceride level	
Normal	<150
Borderline High	150-199
High	200-499

Low-Density Lipoproteins

LDLs are considered the bad form of cholesterol because elevated levels of LDL are associated with greater risk of CVD. LDLs transport highly concentrated amounts of cholesterol to the arterial wall where the cholesterol participates in plaque formation. Because LDLs are the primary plaque-causing lipoprotein, they are the focus of cholesterol/lipid-lowering efforts.

High-Density Lipoproteins

HDL-cholesterol is an independent predictor of coronary heart disease. As the level of HDL increases, the incidence of CVD decreases and visa versa. For every 1-mg/dL decrease in HDL, there is a 3- to 4-percent increase in coronary artery disease.[27]

As HDL-cholesterol decreases (from 60 to 41 to 37), the risk for coronary heart disease increases at all levels of total cholesterol. Additionally, the presence of diabetes or smoking greatly affects the risk associated with a given level of total cholesterol. Hence, a nondiabetic smoker with elevated blood pressure (134/86); an HDL of 41, and a total cholesterol level of 240 to 79 mg/dL has an approximate 20-percent risk of coronary heart disease within 10 years. On the other hand, a diabetic smoker with the same total cholesterol level (240 to 279 mg/dL) but with higher blood pressure (146/94) and a lower HDL-cholesterol has an approximate 45-percent risk of coronary heart disease in the same time period.[28]

Benefits of Improved Lipid Profiles. The risk of CVD decreases when cholesterol levels are reduced. A lowering of total cholesterol by 10 percent reduces the risk of coronary heart disease by 15 percent, and a lowering of LDL-cholesterol by 10 percent reduces the risk of coronary heart disease by approximately 20 percent.[29] Furthermore, treatment that is continued for more than 5 years results in a 25-percent reduction in coronary heart disease events.

Thus, it is critically important that individuals with high cholesterol aggressively pursue treatment (including lifestyle modifications and prescription medications) and that they continue with the treatment plan. It is difficult to overstate the importance of this last point, as too many individuals are tempted to discontinue treatment because the benefits are not obvious to them in the way they feel. That is to say, they may not feel differently when they are on or off medication. Nonetheless, left untreated high cholesterol (especially elevated LDL-cholesterol) is associated with significantly greater rates of death from CVD.

Strategies for Improving Lipid Profiles. The lifetime risk of coronary heart disease can be reduced by 50 percent or more if blood cholesterol levels are reduced before age 40, and 30 percent if reduction in blood cholesterol occurs before 50.[30] The strategies to reduce the risk of CVD associated with dyslipidemia are varied and often overlapping. Furthermore, the degree of risk, and the appropriate interventions, depends on the specific lipid abnormality and the magnitude of the abnormality. In general, the strategies for managing lipid/cholesterol levels fall into two categories: life-style modification and drug therapy. If you have elevated cholesterol, LDLs, or triglycerides, or if you have low HDL levels you should consult a physician to see which combination of strategies is right for you.

Lifestyle Modifications. The primary lifestyle modifications to treat dyslipidemia involve diet and exercise:

- **Diet.** An appropriate diet is an important factor in the prevention and management of dyslipidemia. In general, there are three primary objectives of diet modification for attaining healthy lipid profiles:
  1. Attaining ideal body weight.
  2. Obtaining a well-balanced diet high in fruits and vegetables.
  3. Restricting saturated fats and simple, refined carbohydrates (sugars).[31]

- **Less** than 30 percent of calories should be from fats (with <10 percent of calories coming from saturated fats). Cholesterol intake should be less than 300 mg day. Additionally, there is growing evidence that Omega-3 fatty acids protect against cardiovascular disease, and for that reason it is now recommended commonly that individuals try to eat fish one or two times per week.

- **Exercise.** Exercise is an important component of any weight loss program and weight loss is associated with positive changes in lipid profiles. Furthermore, regular aerobic exercise is associated with decreased triglyceride levels and increased HDL levels.

- **Drug therapy.** Drug therapy may be necessary for individuals who are at high risk for cardiovascular disease (LDLs >160 mg/dL and other risk factors). In all cases, drug therapy should occur in conjunction with dietary therapy and increased physical activity. Prescription drugs are available to treat different lipid disorders (elevated cholesterol, elevated LDLs, low HDLs). In many instances, drug treatment for cholesterol/lipid levels is a long-term treatment strategy, and it is imperative that individuals continue to take their medication. Very often individuals will not "feel better" when they are taking the medication, but the cardiovascular system is "working better." If you have high cholesterol/lipid levels you should follow the diet and exercise guidelines detailed above, take your medicine religiously, and consult with your physician regularly.

Risk Associated with Obesity

Despite what seems to be an obsession with thinness and dieting, approximately 33 percent of the adult population in the United States is obese and another 30 to 35 percent of the population is overweight.[32] The trend in both the adult and the child population toward obesity is increasing. Obesity is associated with a number of diseases, including CVD (high blood pressure, dyslipidemia), diabetes, gallbladder disease, and cancer. Obesity is associated with several other risk factors, but it also exerts an independent influence on the risk of CVD.

As excess body weight (Body Mass Index (BMI)) increases, so does the risk of CVD (Figure B-6).

This relationship is sometimes referred to as a J-shaped curve because, although there is little or no change in mortality at the lower end of the BMI range, as BMI increases above 25, risk begins to increase and does so in a nonlinear fashion. Thus, each incremental pound gained is associated with additional risk for the person who is overweight.

Not only is excess body weight an important risk factor for CVD, but where the weight is carried (fat distribution) is also predictive of heart disease. Abdominal fat increases one's risk of heart disease. This risk can be assessed easily by measuring waist circumference: values greater than 40 inches for males and greater than 35 inches for females indicate an increased risk of heart disease.

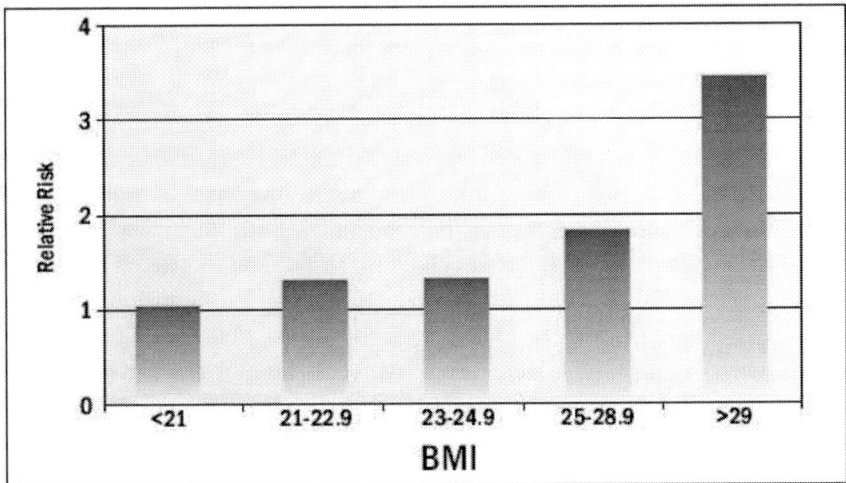

Source: Manson et al. A Prospective Study of Obesity and Risk of Coronary Heart Disease in Women. New England Journal of Medicine. 322:882-889, 1990.

Figure B-6. Relationship Between BMI and Relative Risk of CVD.[33]

- BMI = Wt(kg)/Ht(m)^2
- Assume: Wt = 220 lb, Ht = 5'10"
- Steps
    1. Convert wt to kg by dividing by 2.2 (1 kg = 2.2 lb)
        220/2.2 = 100 kg
    2. Convert height to meters by:
        a. Convert inches to centimeters by multiplying by 2.54
           (1" = 2.54 cm)
           70 x 2.54 = 177 cm
        b. Convert cm to m by dividing by 100 (1 m = 100 cm)
           177 cm = 1.77 m

Plug numbers into formula BMI = 100/1.77^2 = 100/3.13 = 31.9

Figure B-7. Calculation of Body Mass Index (BMI).

Obesity is associated with an increased amount of lipids and cholesterol in the blood. Thus, the LDLs are more likely to invade the arterial wall and initiate plaque development. Obesity also is associated with an inability to utilize carbohydrates causing blood sugar levels to increase. The increased blood glucose levels (and accompanying high levels of insulin) interfere with the ability of the artery to change size (vasodilate) when the heart needs additional blood flow.

The extent of body fatness can be measured in several ways; the most precise laboratory methods involve sophisticated equipment such as underwater weighing tanks or whole body scanning. More commonly, percent body fat is estimated by measuring skinfold thickness at various sites and calculating percent body fat based on the known relationship between skinfold thickness and total body fat. The easiest way, however, to gain a sense of body fatness is through the calculation of BMI (Figure B-7).

This method requires only that height and weight (in meters and kilograms, respectively) be known. Because of its simplicity, the BMI is often used in large-scale studies where hundreds or thousands of people are studied. This simple calculation, however, may overestimate the fatness of some individuals, especially those who are very muscular. Those individuals with a high BMI who do not believe they are overweight or obese, might consult a fitness expert to have percent body fat measured more accurately.

Even modest weight loss can have an important impact on several health parameters, including improvements in blood pressure, lipid profiles, and glucose tolerance.

Strategies for Weight Loss. The strategies to reduce the risk of CVD associated with obesity may seem straightforward: you need to increase the number of calories expended by physical activity (exercise program) and/or you need to decrease the number of calories consumed. Despite what may seem like simple logic, millions of people fail at weight loss attempts each year. In general it is healthful and most likely to be successful if your weight loss program includes a moderate increase in activity and a moderate decrease in caloric intake. Furthermore, you should recognize that your excess weight was not gained in a few weeks or months, and hence you should not try to lose the excess fat in a few weeks or months. Rather, commit yourself to a lifestyle change that you can sustain.

Diet. An appropriate diet is essential to appropriate weight loss. There is considerable controversy over what type of diet is best. In general, it is best to avoid fad diets and stick to proven and healthy diets (i.e., the American Heart Association diet). Your goals should be to:

- attain a healthy body weight;
- eat a well-balanced diet high in fruits and vegetables;
- restrict saturated fats and simple, refined carbohydrates (sugars); and
- eat approximately 250 to 500 calories fewer than you expend each day.

Most experts agree that you should limit your fat intake to less than 30 percent of total calories (with <10 percent of calories coming from saturated fats). Cholesterol intake should be less than 300 mg/day. Additionally, there is growing evidence that Omega-3 fatty acids are protective against CVD, and for that reason, it is now commonly recommended that you try to eat fish one or two times per week.

Exercise is a key part of any weight-loss program. Studies have shown consistently that exercise is particularly effective in maintaining weight loss. Additionally, exercise is the best way to lose fat and maintain muscle mass. When a person loses weight through exercise alone he/she loses fat and muscle. It is the fat that is detrimental to health. In fact, for a firefighter the loss of muscle mass may affect performance negatively because of the high strength demands of the job.

Risk Associated with Type Ii Diabetes

Diabetes is a metabolic disorder characterized by the inability to use sugar (glucose) effectively. In nondiabetic individuals, blood glucose levels increase following the ingestion of carbohydrates (complex sugars) or simple sugar. Increased levels of glucose cause the body to release insulin (a pancreatic hormone), which helps transport glucose from the blood stream into the cells of the body where the glucose is used to make energy or is stored as fuel for later use. Individuals with Type II diabetes tend to have high insulin levels because their cells are resistant to the effects of insulin (a condition known as insulin resistance). Thus the pancreas continues to produce insulin in an attempt to move glucose into the cell. Since insulin is not effective, however, diabetics cannot effectively transport glucose from the blood stream into the cells of the body. Thus, diabetics have high glucose levels in the blood (hyperglycemia).

People with diabetes are twice as likely to experience cardiac events as other individuals. Furthermore, 65 percent of all deaths among diabetic patients are from CVD.[34] As seen in Figure B-8, the degree of cardiovascular risk (and risk of death from all-cause mortality) is directly related to fasting blood glucose levels.[35] Additionally, individuals who have diabetes along with other risk factors are at a much higher risk than nondiabetic individuals with the same number of risk factors.

High blood glucose levels (hyperglycemia) are associated with damage to the smallest blood vessels (such as those in the retina of the eye) and enhanced atherosclerosis. High insulin levels also are associated with enhanced blood clotting.[36]

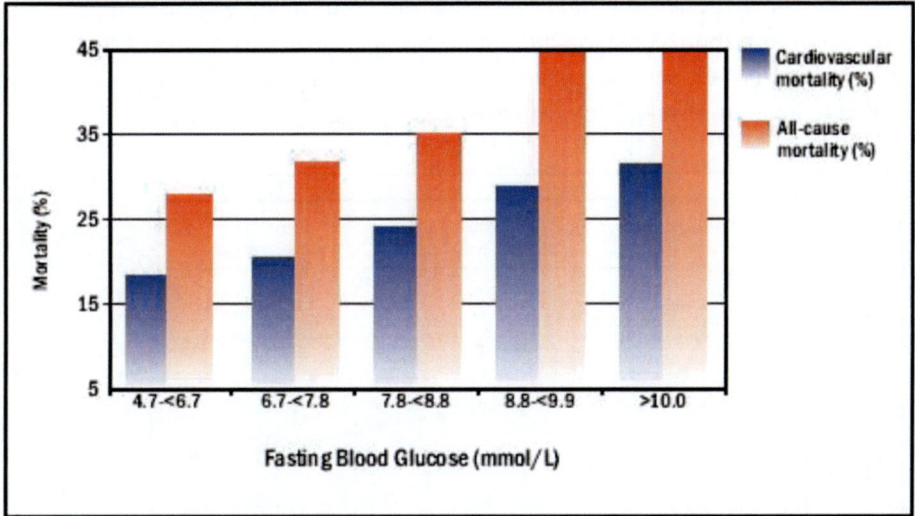

Adapted from: Nesto & Libby. In: Braunwald, Zipes, & Libby. Heart Disease: A Textbook
of Cardiovascular Medicine. 6th Ed. Volume 2. Page 2138.

Figure B-8. Fasting Blood Glucose Levels and Cardiovascular Mortality in Type II
Diabetes Patients.

Strategies for Decreasing Blood Glucose Levels. Diabetes often coexists
with other risk factors for CVD. In fact, the cluster of risk factors has been termed
metabolic syndrome X, and includes abdominal obesity, hypertension,
dyslipidemia, and an inability to use glucose effectively (diabetes). Therefore, it is
important that a person with diabetes very aggressively control other risk factors.
A diabetic should lose excess body weight, exercise regularly, and eat a diet low
in simple sugars and carbohydrates. Because of the complexity of the disease, its
relationship to heart disease, and the difficulty controlling blood glucose levels, a
diabetic person should consult regularly with his/her physician about a diet and
exercise program and the need for medication.

Risk Associated with Physical Inactivity

Physical inactivity is related to several of the risk factors discussed
previously. A lack of exercise increases an individual's risk of obesity,
hypertension, dyslipidemia, and diabetes. However, physical inactivity is also an
independent risk factor for cardiovascular disease. The risk of CVD in inactive
people is about twice that of physically active individuals—approximately the

same as for hypertension and dyslipidemia.[37] In fact, physical inactivity is responsible for approximately 200,000 deaths per year in the United States.[38] As seen in Figure B-9, several studies have shown that CVD mortality is inversely related to level of physical activity or fitness.[39]

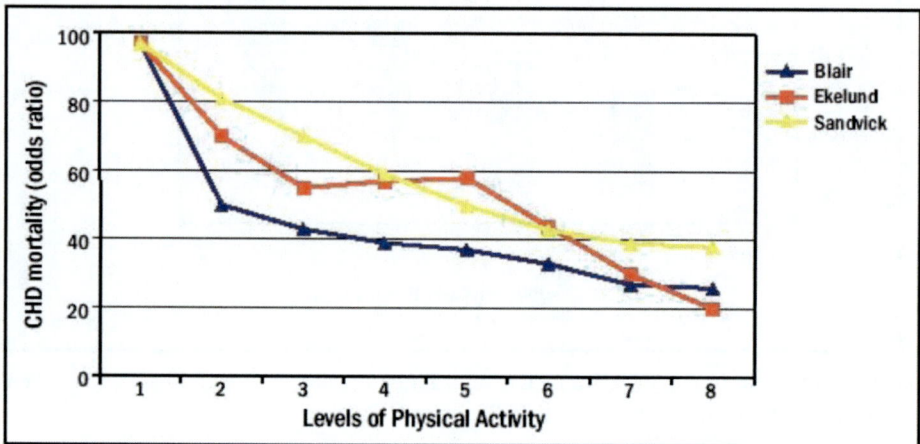

Adapted from: Haskell, et al. Medicine and Science in Sports and Excercise. 26(6), 649-660.

Figure B-9. Relationship Between Physical Activity and Cardiovascular Mortality.[40]

Table B-6. Recommendations for Decreasing CVD Risk Factors

Recommendations	Description
Exercise Moderately	• Decreased blood pressure • Improved lipid (cholesterol) profile • Decreased body fat • Improved glucose tolerance • Eliminates physical inactivity
Eat a Balanced Diet	• Improved lipid (cholesterol) profile • Decreased body weight • Improved glucose tolerance • May decrease blood pressure
Do not Smoke	• Decreased artery blockage • Increased lung health; capacity

Increased physical activity improves work capacity, increases strength, decreases injury rates, and improves heat tolerance. Exercise training also has a positive impact on several other CVD risk factors; it decreases blood pressure, increases HDL, improves glucose tolerance, and causes loss of fat weight. In addition to these substantial benefits, exercise also strengthens the heart muscle, enhances the blood-dissolving capacity of the blood (making unwanted clots less likely), and stabilizes the electrical activity of the heart.

Decreasing Cardiovascular Disease Risk Factors

CVD is a major threat to the health and safety of firefighters. In order to stay healthy, and address the risk factors for developing CVD, a firefighter should adopt a few healthy lifestyle habits. In short, to reduce the risk of suffering a heart attack or stroke, it is imperative that firefighters:

- do not smoke/stop smoking;
- follow a regimen of moderate aerobic exercise; and
- eat a balanced diet, avoiding excess saturated fats, excess simple sugars, and maintaining normal body weight.

Table B-6 summarizes these recommendations and indicates the risk factors that are influenced by each recommendation. Of particular note is the benefit of physical activity in eliminating or favorably affecting five of the six modifiable risk factors.

ACKNOWLEDGEMENTS

The National Volunteer Fire Council (NVFC) Health and Wellness Project, supported by the United States Fire Administration (USFA), was developed to improve health and wellness within the volunteer fire and emergency services. TriData, a Division of System Planning Corporation, assisted the NVFC in developing the Guide.

This study of the current state of health and wellness programs would not have been possible without the cooperation and assistance of many members of the fire service throughout the United States. A number of fire departments are featured throughout the Guide. The NVFC thanks them for their contributions and insights.

The NVFC gratefully acknowledges the USFA for its support in creating this Guide. Additionally, the NVFC would like to recognize the following individuals for their technical assistances with the project:

- *Dr. Denise Smith,* Professor of Exercise Science at Skidmore College and Research Associate at the Illinois Fire Service Institute, offered many hours of technical advice on the Guide and its proposed program. Dr. Smith was a prime contributor to Chapter III (Importance of Health and Wellness for the Volunteer Fire Service) and the author of Appendix B (The Relationship Between Cardiovascular Risk Factors and Physical Fitness).

- *Mr. Fabio Comana,* formerly Exercise Physiologist, Nutritionist, and Wellness Director with Club One Pro Services, Inc., assisted in developing the proposed program as well as alternatives for motivating firefighters to participate in health and wellness programs.

- *Ms. Vicki Lee,* Program Manager at the International Association of Fire Chiefs (IAFC), explained the "Joint-Labor Management Wellness Initiative" and offered insight on implementation of a volunteer program.

At TriData, Patricia Frazier was Project Manager. Ms. Frazier was assisted by Jason Reimer and other members of the TriData staff. Philip Schaenman, President of TriData, provided technical and corporate oversight.

NATIONAL VOLUNTEER FIRE COUNCIL MISSION STATEMENT

To provide a unified voice for volunteer Fire/EMS organizations.
This Mission will be accomplished by:

- Representing the interests of the volunteer Fire/EMS organizations at the U.S. Congress and federal agencies.
- Promoting the interests of the state and local organizations at the national level.
- Promoting and providing education and training for the volunteer Fire/EMS organizations.

- Providing representation on national standards setting committees and projects.

Gathering information from and disseminating information to the volunteer Fire/EMS organizations.

End Notes

[1] Phillips, Jack, et al. The Human Resources Scorecard. 2000.
[2] United States Fire Administration. *Fire and Emergency Medical Services Ergonomics–A Guide for Understanding and Implementing An Ergonomics Program in Your Department.*
[3] Heron, et al. "Deaths: Final Data for 2004."
[4] United States Fire Administration, *Firefighter Fatality Retrospective Study.* Apr. 2002.
[5] Ibid.
[6] Karter and Molis. "Firefighter Injuries for 2006."
[7] United States Fire Administration, *Firefighter Fatality Retrospective Study.*
[8] Fahy, Rita, and Paul Leblanc. "Firefighter Fatalities 2001." *NFPA Journal.* July/August 2002.
[9] Ibid.
[10] Centers for Disease Control and Prevention, *Annual Smoking-Attributable Mortality.*
[11] Ibid.
[12] Ridker, Genest, and Libby, Op. cit.
[13] Plowman and Smith, Op. cit.
[14] *The Health Benefits of Smoking Cessation.* A Report from the Surgeon General. 1990.
[15] Ridker, Genest, and Libby, Op. cit.
[16] Kaplan, Op. cit.
[17] National High Blood Pressure Education Program Working Group. *Arch. Intern Med.,* 1993.
[18] Ridker, Genest, and Libby, Op. cit.
[19] Kaplan, Op. cit.
[20] Ibid.
[21] Ibid.
[22] Oberman, Op. cit.
[23] Gaziano, Mason, and Ridker, Op. cit.
[24] Ibid.
[25] Oberman, Op. cit.
[26] Summary of the Third Report of the National Cholesterol Education Program. 2001.
[27] Gaziano, Mason, and Ridker, Op. cit.
[28] Oberman, Op. cit.
[29] Ibid.
[30] Ibid.
[31] Ridker, Genest, and Libby, Op. cit.
[32] Ogden, Carroll, Curtin, McDowell, Tabak, and Flegal, Op. cit.
[33] Manson, et al. Op. cit.
[34] American Diabetes Association, Op. cit.
[35] Nesto and Libby, Op. cit.
[36] Ridker, Genest, and Libby, Op. cit.
[37] Plowman and Smith, Op. cit.
[38] Ridker, Genest, and Libby, Op. cit.
[39] Haskell, Op. cit.
[40] Ibid.

CHAPTER SOURCES

The chapters included in this book have been previously published as edited, excerpted and augmented editions of a United States Fire Administration, Health and Wellness Guide for the Volunteer Fire and Emergency Services, dated February 2009.

INDEX